Physician Empowerment through Capitation

Clifford R. Frank, MHSA
President
Healthcare Management Solutions, Inc.
Jacksonville, Florida

and

I. David Kibbe, MBA
President
Excellence in Health Care
Clifton, Virginia

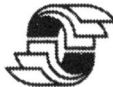

AN ASPEN PUBLICATION®
Aspen Publishers, Inc.
Gaithersburg, Maryland
2000

Library of Congress Cataloging-in-Publication Data

Frank, Clifford R.
Physician empowerment through capitation / Clifford R. Frank, I. David Kibbe.
p. cm.
Includes index.
ISBN 0-86421-212-9
1. Capitation fees (Medical care)   I. Kibbe, I. David.   II. Title.
R728.6.F72 2000
362.1'068'1—dc21
99-052792

Orders: (800) 638-8437
Customer Service: (800) 234-1660

About Aspen Publishers • For more than 40 years, Aspen has been a leading professional publisher in a variety of disciplines. Aspen's vast information resources are available in both print and electronic formats. We are committed to providing the highest quality information available in the most appropriate format for our customers. Visit Aspen's Internet site for more information resources, directories, articles, and a searchable version of Aspen's full catalog, including the most recent publications: **http://www.aspenpublishers.com**
Aspen Publishers, Inc. • The hallmark of quality in publishing
Member of the worldwide Wolters Kluwer group.

Editorial Services: Nora Fitzpatrick
Library of Congress Catalog Card Number: 99-052792
ISBN: 0-8342-1212-9

Printed in the United States of America

1 2 3 4 5

TABLE OF CONTENTS

CONTRIBUTORS

Editors

Clifford R. Frank, MHSA
President
Healthcare Management
Solutions, Inc.
Jacksonville, Florida

I. David Kibbe, MBA
President
Excellence in Health Care
Clifton, Virginia

Contributors

Bruce Ardis, MBA
Principal
Ardis Group
Columbia, Maryland

Jon A. Brunsberg, MBA
Principal
Reden & Anders, Ltd.
Minneapolis, Minnesota

Fred C. Campbell, Jr., MD,
FACP
Clinical Professor of Medicine
U.T. Health Science Center
San Antonio, Texas

Timothy M. Davlantes, MD
Chief Medical Consultant
Healthcare Management
Solutions, Inc.
Jacksonville, Florida

Joel Hornberger, MHS
Chief Operating Officer
Cherokee Health Systems
Talbott, Tennessee

David C. Main, Esq.
Partner
Shaw Pittman
Washington, DC

T. Lane Macalester, Esq.
Counsel
Shaw Pittman
Washington, DC

Steven R. Peskin, MD, MBA, FACP
President/Chief Operating Officer
NCI Managed Care
Princeton, New Jersey

Debi Reissman, Pharm.D.
President
Rxperts
Irvine, California

Jonothan C. Tierce, C. Phil.
Principal
Epinomics Research Inc.
Arlington, Virginia

Lynette L. Trygstad, FSA
Principal
Reden & Anders, Ltd.
Minneapolis, Minnesota

PREFACE

Capitation as a payment system for medical care has waxed and waned over the last decade. Capitation has worked well in some environments, horribly in others. The chief lesson over the last decade has been that if capitation is forced onto a community of practitioners, it usually doesn't work well. But if practitioners see clinical improvements and financial advantage, capitation can be a useful mechanism to align incentives throughout the health care process. Capitation cannot substitute for sound clinical judgment. Nor is capitation automatically at cross-purposes to high quality care. Just as fee-for-service systems are open to abuse, capitated systems require clinical oversight to ensure care is appropriately provided.

This book is designed to speak to the reader who is familiar with capitation basics, but not deeply experienced in the operational, institutional, and administrative complications involved in capitated care. The book often speaks in the voices of experience—experiences of pain, learning, resilience, and triumph. The cases are told from personal perspectives that give the reader an inside glimpse into the intense political and organizational challenges posed by capitation. The results have not always been pretty or neat, but the experiences these authors bring highlight important competencies that individuals and organizations need to master before the learning curve overwhelms the participants.

Why do practitioners engage in capitated contracts? The answers change with each business setting, but fall into five general categories: (1) to provide a steady cashflow, (2) to lock-in or capture new patients (market share), (3) to control clinical decision making, (4) to eliminate the fear of being left out or abandoned by patients and payers, and (5) to just sign any contract. Whatever the reason, the reality is usually different than what was expected initially. This book is designed to provide the reader with real situations that can serve as the basis for a realistic understanding of what it takes to succeed in a capitated world.

But the world isn't going capitated this month. The underlying economic pressures to contain health care costs have not changed, and premium trends strongly suggest greater economic pressures coming soon. Having the choice of practitioners was great when it was free. But as premiums rise, time and again we have seen patients trade choice for price. Several alternate models are already in the market that either limit premium or limit choice. New capitated models such as contact capitation allow plans to offer both reasonable premiums and a broad choice of practitioners. As these new capitation models become more common, the capitated market will grow. The link between economic alignment and clinical behavior is too strong to ignore, and too powerful not to harness.

This book covers the business aspects of capitation while providing each reader a set of experiences that make real the challenges of doing capitation right. The first chapter lays out the case for why capitation will continue, in one form or another, as a payment system in the future. Market forces are at work continually reshaping the health care delivery and financing system, and the most efficient economic model cannot be long ignored by insurers, businesses, and policymakers.

In the next chapters, the contributing authors explore the difficulties and adaptive strategy employed in managing care in a capitated system. The turnaround case illustrates the wide variety of moving parts within a capitated care system, and the difficulty in making those parts move in harmony. The contact capitation case presents the difficulty of implementing innovations in a large, multispecialty IPA/PHO with all the inherent conflicting interests and agendas of the parties.

The interview with a seasoned capitated physician working with a primarily Medicare HMO population identifies key differences between capitated and fee-for-service mindsets. The specialty capitation case identifies administrative hazards posed by capitated specialty carve-out arrangements that painful experience has taught.

The capitated Medicaid case illustrates the special challenges posed by government programs run by executive fiat and provides insight into the internal organizational havoc caused by the external pressures.

Pharmacy, risk distribution, incurred-but-not-reported claims analysis, and legal issues are presented to give the reader a sense of these important dimensions of capitated programs.

The Bootcamp section of this book is designed for the capitation beginner. This section provides vignettes about capitation and the various trials, traps, and triumphs of the trade. The book can be read straight through, or readers can hop around to topics that best fit their immediate needs. Either way, the lessons remain, and the stories are no less compelling.

We hope that you take away from each visit with this book a little of the excitement and some of the cautions laid before you.

Clifford R. Frank, MHSA
I. David Kibbe, MBA

PART I

Frontline Stories of the
Pain and Gain of Capitation

CHAPTER 1

Market Opportunities Still Abound for Capitation

Clifford R. Frank, MHSA, and I. David Kibbe, MBA

Capitation as a health maintenance organization (HMO) payment mechanism to physicians and hospitals has been battered by a series of major missteps including the bankruptcy of FPA Medical Management, MedPartners' withdrawal from the physician management business, and the general market movement toward broader patient access to physicians. But, just as the HMO industry survived the Maxicare bankruptcy in the 1980s, managed care will find new applications for capitation concepts. The market is not static. The market for health care services and financing is comprised of significantly differing segments that move at different speeds, in different directions, for different reasons. It is this market diversity that prevents a one-size-fits-all business model from consolidating the physician services industry. The market diversity also ensures that capitation will be a factor in the health services market for many years to come. Capitation answers market needs.

As of this writing, global capitation including institutional risk is still a significant factor in many markets, provider networks, and medical groups. Global capitation, when managed well and funded fairly can yield substantial rewards to network participants. Global capitation when underfunded, or undermanaged, can suck the lifeblood out of contracting providers in a relatively short period of time.

In some markets, such as in the upper Midwest, global professional capitation with institutional gain sharing is a successful payment model. In other markets, such as California, a transition away from global capitation is underway, triggered by underfunded capitation rates that have eroded the financial base of many provider groups. In South Florida, the dominant risk-sharing model has been single specialty capitation, but that model is currently under stress as well. Capitation is not a cure for low premiums. Capitation can help stabilize premiums and create a basis for redesigning patient care processes to deliver a better product. When capitation is used to beat up providers, quality of care can suffer. Network instability follows and eventually may prompt intervention by the State Insurance Commissioner.

SINGLE SPECIALTY CAPITATION GROWING

As the authors write this book, risk contracting is changing from vertical provider system global capitation arrangements to more horizontal single specialty networks. Payers originally moved en masse to global capitation arrangements as a means of cushioning earnings' fluctuations to please Wall Street. HMO stock companies found that Wall Street's penalty for missing quarterly earnings targets was too great. HMOs moved to global capitation arrangements across many markets and products, often without assessing the providers' capacity for absorbing and managing the risk for which they were contracting. The HMO operational imperative was to shift risk to providers to smooth the quarterly earnings announcements.

Single specialty capitation has moved to the forefront of payer contract strategies for three reasons. First, single specialty contracting dilutes the network power of large health systems and their affiliated medical staff. The single specialty approach offers physicians the potential of market gain and may even offer facility savings bonuses for their specialty services. The upside to payers can be substantial by transferring outpatient procedures from hospital outpatient departments to lower cost freestanding centers combined with physicians finding alternate treatments for marginal cases. Those savings can approach a 30–50 percent reduction in specialty costs over current experience.

The second reason why specialty capitation contracting is attractive to payers is that the effort can be focused on the real network problem areas instead of just a broad recontracting effort that creates substantial physician market resistance. By focusing on specialties that are cost outliers on a per member per month (pmpm) basis, payers can fix the right problem. This was the logic used when payers moved to mental health capitation carve-outs. Now, specialty capitation has moved mainstream to include cardiology, ophthalmology, urology, ENT, and many other specialties. Each market has its own anomalies and quirks. Specialty capitation allows a payer to mold its contracting strategies to market aberrations as it sees fit, rather than turning the whole premium and reward for effectively managing utilization over to a globally capitated entity.

A third attraction of specialty capitation contracting is the prospect of providers winnowing the network of high-utilizing physicians, rather than the payer having to narrow the network at some legal risk. By recontracting the specialty network, payers can avoid many of the legal risks associated with physician termination. Knowledgeable providers will select physicians who exhibit conservative clinical practice profiles so as to be able to function effectively on a capitated basis.

Payers are, however, more acutely aware that dumping a risk contract— even a single specialty risk contract—on an ill-prepared network poses market and financial risks back onto the payer. If the single specialty network fails, the payer may end up bearing the risk, the financial cost of a bailout, and the cost of bad publicity that accompanies such a catastrophe. Employers now expect payers to adequately credential the networks with which payers subcontract care. Such employer expectations of payers also extend to provider network oversight, compliance with the National Committee for Quality Assurance (NCQA), and the Health Plan Employer Data and Information Set (HEDIS) reporting measures and other regulatory issues. Payers no longer can shift the risk and look the other way when financial implosions occur.

THE MARKET PENDULUM

Capitation as a payer contracting strategy has historically ebbed and flowed depending upon market dynamics, perceived utilization savings opportunities, and premium trends. When payers could make money without shifting risk, they chose not to do so. As premium trends leveled and Wall Street pressures for no earnings surprises mounted, payers looked more favorably on capitated arrangements. Currently, premium trends are moving upward, and payers want the benefit of those added monies. Capitation agreements are breaking under the weight of increasing utilization, weak provider capitation infrastructure, market demands for greater choice of providers, and increasing regulatory requirements for capital reserves by risk contracting organizations. All these forces are moving the market toward unwinding global capitation arrangements in many areas. But, such movements also create countermovements within markets. Single specialty capitation, direct payer capitation of specialists through targeted specialty budgets, and new episode of care payment systems are all attempts to move beyond dysfunctional capitation systems currently in place. Signs also point to other market dynamics that can be expected to create new demands for capitated care within the next three years.

Unit costs, premium costs, and administrative costs drive the pendulum of the market. The current premium cost trends are moving up toward double digits. These premium trend factors are loaded into the health insurance premiums employers must pay for employer-sponsored health insurance. Employers can hop from payer to payer to miss one year's rate increase. (But payers move en masse on pricing, but the timing from one payer to another may vary slightly.) Insurers must file their rates with state insurance departments with the result that most insurers, HMOs, preferred provider organizations (PPOs), and self-insured employers know what pricing effects are sweeping the market. They have a window into their competitors' pricing practices through these state rate filings. When a major payer in a market decides that they have lost enough money chasing market share, they raise rates. Others then follow suit knowing that most employers will not switch carriers so long as the rate increase is within market norms. This underwriting cycle takes place about every six to seven years with three favorable years of profitable underwriting followed by three or four unfavorable years. The market is going through one of these swings now, and will continue to do so for the next two to three years.

What is different about this cycle is that employers face a special challenge in this robust economy. Employers have little pricing power in that they cannot pass through cost increases to their customers without suffering substantial business losses. But, employers also face a tough labor market, meaning they are reluctant to pass premium cost increases through to employees for fear of suffering employee recruiting and retention problems. What seems to be happening in most markets across the country is that employers are taking the HMO premium increases in the first year of the upward trend in the underwriting cycle, but their behavior in Year 2 and Year 3 is open to speculation.

NEW PRODUCTS FROM HMOs

Many HMOs are betting that employers will want more creative alternatives than these two ugly choices—passing through premium increases to customers or passing through premium increases to employees. One alternative that many HMOs have recently initiated is to develop separate products geared toward either specific provider systems or especially efficient providers who can deliver a lower utilization level and therefore a lower price to employers and employees. These new subnetwork products are in some cases coming at the behest of larger employers wanting to move their employees into more cost-effective systems. In other cases these efforts are sponsored by coalitions of small businesses looking to have a market impact. In either case, the effect is the same. Employees will be offered a whole new set of benefit plans that are less expensive than other choices, but that also include fewer physicians, hospitals, and options for choice.

Choice is a characteristic most of us value, but to differing degrees. Broadening patient choice has been a marketing mantra for the last five years in managed care as premiums stabilized and, in some cases, moved down. Employees clamored for more physician and hospital choice, and managed care networks became more inclusive rather than less. So long as choice was cost free, employees demanded it. HMOs with smaller, tighter networks were punished in the market as larger network products priced at the same premium level gained market share. But, the cost management side of the business failed to keep pace with product growth, resulting in HMO deficits, earnings surprises, staff layoffs, and acquisitions/mergers. Now premiums are rising, and employees will not happily pay additional premiums for the broad networks they now enjoy.

Broad network premium differentials could easily approach 20–30 percent within two years as actuaries work in the costs associated with member selection and retention, clinical cost savings in smaller networks, and the benefits of capitating providers in narrower networks. Providers will find that the broad network contracts and fee schedules they now enjoy will deteriorate both in volume and price level. Fee schedules will be cut within broad network products to support product-pricing requirements. And patient volumes in these broad network products will diminish as the premium costs are passed to employees, and they choose more narrow products at lower out-of-pocket costs. The cycle of the early 1990s is likely to repeat.

For efficient, knowledgeable providers, entering capitation contracts as the premium cycle accelerates is good market timing. Capitated providers will be in a position to harvest enrollment gains as patients migrate from higher cost, broad access plans to more narrowly focused HMO products that are more affordable. Employers will likely tie their employee contribution to the lowest cost insurance product.

CHANGES IN GOVERNMENT PROGRAMS

The opportunities evident in commercial HMO populations may also be present in government programs including Medicare and Medicaid. Government programs have tended to follow rather than lead commercial managed care programs in design and implementation of new products and methods. The health care cost control pressures that face state and federal agencies remain. The drift toward managed care may slow for a period, but budget pressures and a commercial surge in new product development will rekindle government's interest in expanding managed care offerings to Medicare and Medicaid beneficiaries. The initial attempts at expanding provider-sponsored organization contracting opportunities have proven less fruitful than hoped, but the budgetary squeeze is only going to grow in the future. As the population ages, Medicare spending will continue to increase, thereby increasing the attractiveness of a managed care solution to policymakers. Capitation in one form or another will likely be a part of such a solution because the economics are so compelling. The standard Medicare population uses hospital resources at the rate of 2,500 inpatient days per 1,000 Medicare beneficiaries per year. Take that same population and put them in a well-run capitated program and their hospital days per 1,000 will drop to less than 900. A system that uses 60 percent less of the most expensive health care resource while keeping patients healthy and satisfied cannot be ignored. Policymakers will not ignore capitated systems of care as they look for alternatives to exploding budgets and huge downstream cost increases. Capitation will be part of the solution set for Medicare. What form and who will control the particulars is open to debate. But, the economic imperative will ultimately drive the system components toward a capitated solution among several heterogeneous approaches.

CAPITATION NOW AND IN THE FUTURE

Capitation contracting continues to evolve and respond to market demands. Physicians and hospitals will continue to pursue reliable revenue streams in order to spread their fixed costs across a larger base of patients. Payers in search of new products, new structures, and new marketing opportunities will continue to ponder alternatives that contain costs and provide adequate access to meet the needs of various market segments.

Somewhere in the middle, payers and providers will periodically find each other and develop business arrangements that work for both parties. Many times those arrangements will include capitation of one form or another. The economic imperatives to contain costs, lock in revenue streams, and serve patients' needs are intertwined with opportunities big and small.

The next chapters highlight cases where capitated provider networks have had to deal with very tough internal issues. While the answers described here do not always translate to other situations, the questions and challenges they pose do.

SUGGESTED READINGS

Haugh, R. 1998. Who's Afraid of Capitation Now? *Hospitals & Health Networks.*

Predictions '99: Solid Year Ahead as Industry Evolves, Finances Stabilize. 1999. *Health Market Survey*, 14 January.

Robinson, J. 1999. The Future of Managed Care Organization. *Health Affairs* 18, No. 2: 7–23.

Chapter 2

Physicians Step Up to the Capitation Challenge

I. David Kibbe, MBA

Don Cheek, Summer Clinic administrator, strode into the staff meeting, his eyes blazing with fury and disgust. "I've just gone over our year-to-date results from the Allcare capitation commercial contract, and they stink! How are we going to present these results to our Executive Committee next week? Sixty-three cents on the dollar compared to what we would have gotten for fee-for-service. That's way below what we had projected when we signed this contract four years ago, and it's headed lower based on your calculations, right?"

His CFO, Penny Kincaid, stared straight ahead as she started to respond. "It's what I've been telling you. We never should have entered into this capitation contract with Allcare. We would have been better off maintaining our fee-for-service business and forgoing the growth. Thirty-five docs and profitable business is a lot better than what we have today."

"Penny, drop it! We can't roll back to the past, and you're disregarding what we gained by this contract and the 35,000 members that we provide care for through it. I sold our physicians on the growth and the long-term positioning in the market. That's what they bought, and that's what we've delivered. We need to focus on making these financials work a lot better, though. I've come this far, and I don't plan to make this contract my professional funeral pyre. Let's push ahead and get things set for the Executive Committee meeting next week. Ok?"

SETTING THE STAGE

Summer Clinic had started up more than 70 years prior to this scene. During most of these many years, it had served as a well-regarded, multispecialty group of 30 physicians. Internal medicine, pediatrics, and medical and surgical subspecialties provided the nucleus of the group, with most emphasis placed on specialty care. The group's governance was dominated by these specialists for years.

Driven by its ambition to establish a cutting edge reputation, Summer Clinic invited Allcare, a Colorado-based managed care company, to establish a joint venture with the medical group. As part of the agreed upon joint venture, Summer Clinic assumed a one-third ownership interest in Allcare Midwest and three positions on a nine-person board. More importantly, it entered into an exclusive five year, percentage-of-premium commercial capitation contract with the managed care company. Allcare delivered on its promise of a strong market entry, at one point becoming the seventh fastest growing health plan in the country. Membership rocketed to 30,000 in three years before growth began to taper off. Summer Clinic met this growth by adding 15 physicians to the group, almost all of them in family practice, to meet the requirements for primary care physicians who were oriented to serving a panel of members. Expanding from one central site, Summer opened four other sites around the city, particularly in areas of rapid growth, to enhance patient access and convenience. Moreover, it responded to explicit demands by Allcare to provide marketable sites or risk losing exclusivity as the plan expanded.

Summer Clinic benefited from a long-standing, albeit tenuous, relationship, with Southside Medical Center, a 600-bed tertiary facility operating in the fastest growing part of the city. Summer's primary central site stood nearby Southside, and a number of its specialists played prominent roles on the center's medical staff. Summer would periodically talk with other hospitals about establishing alternative arrangements, but the force of history, inertia, and quality kept them largely focused on admitting to Southside. At the same time, Summer managed to develop a number of competitive ambulatory capabilities including an outpatient surgery center. Southside responded by acquiring practices and consolidating them into a competing, captive medical group operating nearby. Southside and Summer needed each other, in many ways, but were wary of their mutual dependence, creating an awkward, sometimes hostile relationship.

Several years later, Summer was greeted with the opportunity to take on the management and partial ownership of the struggling Olney IPA (independent practice association) previously affiliated with Northside Medical Center. Summer Clinic saw this as an opportunity to expand its geographic reach, expand its hospital relationships, and spread its overhead costs to the management services organization (MSO) serving the IPA. Moreover, it created the potential for becoming the primary regional physician consolidator and organizer. At the same time, Summer was concerned about the assumption of the IPA due to its declining financial performance and uneven reputation. In the short term, it would create more challenges than opportunities. Olney was a 200-physician IPA, anchored by a dozen primary care physicians with a reasonable track record in managing care for its population of members. Its geographic reach and reputation were particularly strong in the outlying sections of the metropolitan area, which again constituted more rapid growth. Olney IPA, though, had insufficient scale to operate efficiently and lacked influence over a large percentage of its physicians, hence its interest in teaming up with a larger, stronger player like Summer Clinic with complementary geographic coverage.

THE FINANCIAL CHALLENGE

The capitation contract that Summer Clinic and Allcare had initially negotiated was structured to pay Summer 82.6 percent of the commercial premium after deducting the cost of benefit riders that were excluded from the arrangement. Vision, dental, durable medical equipment, and drug costs, for example, were not the responsibility of Summer and hence, the premiums calculated for those benefits were handled outside the calculation of the capitation. Eighty-two and six-tenths percent of the remaining commercial premium then was paid to Summer as its capitation for each member enrolled with the Summer Clinic.

To enable a strong start in the market, Allcare had priced its commercial HMO products aggressively, about 10 percent below the market, generating an average commercial premium of $105 per member per month (pmpm) during its first three years of operation. After deducting benefit riders, the resulting premium, applied to the capitation calculation for Summer was $90 per member per month, resulting in an average capitation of $74.34 pmpm during this period. Summer's service responsibilities included professional medical services, ambulatory care, hospital-based physician services, inpatient hospital, home health care, diagnostics, and skilled nursing facility. Allcare participated in the risk related to hospital and other facility costs on a one-third basis and provided reinsurance above identified limits. Prescription drugs were not included in the capitation or risk pools for Summer Clinic.

The first two years of financial experience generated capitation that was the equivalent of 78 percent of what they believed would have been generated in their previous fee-for-service environment. Given the growing prevalence of discounted fees in managed care contracts, Summer concluded that their capitation revenue was only 5 percent lower than it would have been. Moreover, Allcare had generated the desired revenue and patient growth, enabling the Clinic to spread its fixed costs over a larger base. Additionally, Allcare had agreed to fund initial startup and operational costs related to creating an MSO that Summer would use to manage its contracts. The purchase of software and part of the cost of two clinicians and an HMO coordinator were included in this funding. Low cost financing and guarantees were also provided to Summer to enable its expansion to two additional sites. With this as a base, Summer Clinic looked forward to continued growth in the remaining years of its contract.

The financial picture though began changing rapidly. Inpatient utilization, which had quickly and steadily declined over the first two years, first leveled off and then started to edge up. Its average length of stay for hospitalized patients increased. Hospital-based physician costs jumped by a full dollar per member per month. Ambulatory surgery rates per thousand continued to climb even as inpatient admission rates leveled off. Urgent care and emergency visits increased. Specialty referrals climbed 32 percent. More ominously, referrals to specialists outside Summer Clinic constituted the largest portion of that increase. Out-of-area care increased 20 percent. The incidence of catastrophic cases tripled. The cost per hospital day declined 5 percent for a period following contract negotiation but then increased back to its previous level as the percentage of ICU days to total funds increased by 20 percent. Membership growth slowed to a more normal rate of adding 500 net new members per month and then to half of that by the end of the year.

Further complicating the situation, Allcare's financial support during the preoperational period and first two years of operation began to phase out as membership thresholds were reached. Less financing support was provided for the third and then the fourth sites established by the Clinic. The MSO staff doubled in number to respond to the larger membership and the changing utilization. Premium increases of 7 and 8 percent translated into capitation increases of only 2 percent as an increasing amount of the premium was allocated to soaring drug costs that were outside Summer's responsibility. The cost of recruiting and retaining staff at Summer increased in a tight market. The cost of installing new workstations, networking, and maintaining programs increased, as the administrative complexity of the MSO grew geometrically.

The capitation yield for Summer fell from its satisfactory level of 78 percent of fee-for-service (FFS) equivalency to 72 percent and then 67 percent the following year even as the medical group became increasingly reliant on capitation as a major source of revenue. Specialist physician income leveled off and then declined. Primary care incomes, which needed to increase significantly to recruit the right physicians, instead increased moderately and then stayed at tepid, less competitive levels. Several new physicians stayed less than two years. Others took on an increasing patient load without concomitant rewards and compensation. Patient dissatisfaction with the physician turnover increased. That was exacerbated by comments made by the physicians to their patients about Allcare, its marketing, and its inadequate capitation.

ADDRESSING THE CHALLENGE

Don Cheek sat down awkwardly in his chair at the table, clearly thinking about his financials, not his feet. His staff, for the most part, were competent medical practice personnel who had learned a heck of a lot about insurance and managed care during the past several years. Nonetheless, they still saw the world largely through conventional practice eyes, developed over the years prior to the Allcare contract. In addition to Penny as his CFO, he had Sam Wiley, his Information Systems administrator, Bill Page, as Associate Administrator for Operations, and Deirdre Pace, MSO manager. Altogether, these five key administrative staff had more than 50 years of practice management experience, the vast majority of which predated their current challenge.

Sam chimed in first, "I've just run some reports that I think we would all find useful to review. Wish I had this data sooner, but our conversion to the JIT Cap System took longer than expected, as you know." Sam directed everyone to the third page of the printout, pointing to the "adds and deletes." "Those jerks at Allcare don't know how to market any longer, or they're playing games with us; probably both. What do you think, Penny? You've seen this in the preliminary run that I did. "

Penny wanted to respond in her usual diatribe about managed care generally and Allcare, specifically, but Don had made it clear that wasn't going to go far. "Well, there are a lot of problems here that I see. Our per member per month yield is down due to the increased average contract size. Allcare is selling more family contracts and larger ones at that. I never feel that the number of visits and referrals decreases as much as they say it will due to the presence of healthy children. That's clearly a problem! Our referrals are way up. Dr. Dewitt just changed the review criteria again, right, Deirdre? I've gone over the contract provisions again, particularly the matrix on benefit coverage accountabilities. There is some ambiguity there that we need to address. Related to that, I think that the costs of some of the benefits that they added on were not projected well, leaving us on the short end, again. We are definitely veering off on the high side on the utilization benchmarks that we set last year, in almost all categories. The only good news about the Olney IPA's performance is that it makes us look good. Those guys are a joke."

"Alright, Penny, I appreciate the work that you and Sam have done already in getting this data worked up. It's about time that we at least have this to work with," Don added. "The data are never as good as we'd like, so let's start talking about our alternatives. That's what the Executive Committee will want to hear from me next week. They'll have a bunch of opinions about the cause of this situation, but I want to move past that once they've had their opportunity to vent. No doubt, I'll be a few inches shorter at the end of that, but that's the way it goes in this business. Let's list the alternative actions on the flip pad here."

Action Alternatives:

1. Negotiate an increase in capitation with Allcare.
2. Conduct a detailed audit of enrollment data and pools administered by Allcare.
3. Tighten internal review of referrals.
4. Tighten management of enrollment and disen-rollment.
5. Track and manage complex cases more effectively.
6. Revamp the physician compensation system to discourage utilization.
7. Shift hospital care to less expensive hospitals.
8. Tighten specialty contracting including specialty cap.
9. Implement contact cap with specialists within clinic.
10. Limit growth by closing panels on most PCPs.
11. Shift membership among physicians based on cost performance.
12. Revamp Olney IPA, accelerating its integration into MSO functions.

A DEBATE ENSUES

The following Wednesday, the Summer Clinic Executive Committee meeting convened at 6:10 PM. Five agenda items were noted, but most of the time would be spent on the financials and the Allcare capitation experience. Dr. Jeff Stuart, a 42-year-old family practitioner calmly called the meeting to order. His unflappable demeanor masked his intense drive and focused leadership. Those around the table knew him well, though. Jeff had effectively led a "coup" among the younger primary care physicians resulting in an almost complete overturning of the Clinic physician leadership. Once dominated by 50-year-old-plus specialists with Clinic tenure of more than 20 years each, Summer had turned to a different set during the past two years as it grappled with its growth, its increasing prepaid care, and the necessity for new interventions among partners and employees. Jeff brought a cool directness to his role as Chairman that was not tinged by needless emotion. Moreover, he could be incredibly direct while genuinely seeking input as he established consensus among his colleagues. His political skills were significant.

"Let's get going. We have a lot to go over this evening, particularly the third item on our financial performance. Don, would you give us a management update, first?"

Don laid out the prior month's operating statistics in rapid order. He stopped to field a handful of largely clarifying questions from physician leaders. He then reported on the status of the most recent clinic site opening.

"Southbrook opened 10 days later than planned due to subcontractor work and the late arrival of some equipment. We promoted the opening well and conveyed the change in dates. About 400 Allcare members have transferred to Southbrook and a handful of our FFS patients. We've seen some new traffic there also. Overall, though, we're slower than we expected given the growth on that side of the city, generally. This is consistent with the leveling off in membership growth with Allcare that we've seen over the past months."

"Well, where were you and Allcare on those marketing projections a year ago when we first planned this site?" interrupted Dr. Joe Lugar, an abrupt but highly capable internist. "Couldn't you have foreseen this? I'm tired of bankrolling their potential growth and being on the line for their achieving it! They aren't delivering, and we're left holding the bag."

"Dr. Lugar," Don responded, "we planned this site under three different scenarios, and they all work in the long term. Admittedly, we are behind even the conservative scenario, and that's going to create short-term pressure on us. We did negotiate guarantees with Allcare that will help to protect us in the near term."

"Joe, let's keep going. There are a lot of interwoven elements to discuss; this is just one of them, right? Don, let's finish this off so that we can get to the larger financial issues," Dr. Stuart directed. That said, Don completed the Management Update and asked to lead off the next item, which was the focus of the Executive Committee that evening.

"My staff and I met several times over the past week to review information that we have been able to pull together since completing the conversion of our cap system. To put it succinctly, as we had thought, our financial performance related to the Allcare capitation contract has steadily declined since contract inception, three years ago. Moreover, we expect some further deterioration in the coming months before, I believe, turning it around. We have laid out a number of alternative actions, few of which are exclusive of one another. We simply need to agree on which ones are doable and will give us the biggest bang. Others can follow later once we get the big hits. I'd like to start.

"Don, your optimism may be encouraging to some, but I'm tiring of it, frankly," interrupted Dr. Bill Singer, a urologist and the lone specialist on the Executive Committee. "I wasn't in favor of the Allcare capitation when we started, and I'm sure not now. It's a black hole that is sucking my income and that of many of my colleagues right down a hole. We work harder and harder for less and less money. I joined this group for the opportunity for positive peer interactions, the ease of referrals, the quality of care, and the ability to earn a fair income. I did not join Summer to subsidize a bunch of second-rate physicians in some ill-formed IPA or to make managed care executives millionaires. All we've got now is a three-year downward drift in income, all the while working harder."

"Bill, thank you for sharing that with us again," Dr. Jeff Stuart, responded. "You have defined one end of the spectrum of our alternatives. We can push this to the brink with Allcare. Either they capitulate and revise the contractual terms to our benefit, or we're out of it with 180 days' notice, right? If we go there, we must expect them to dig in their heels. We have a lot of volume at stake here that we have expanded around over the past several years. But let's have Don finish outlining the alternatives before we debate each one separately."

Almost 30 minutes later, Don Cheek wrapped up his review of the details of the capitation results and the 12 alternative actions proposed that he and his staff had worked up. Body language, among the physicians, clearly indicated that the actions most concerning to them related to compensation system changes and increased cost and utilization performance scrutiny. Changes in hospital admitting patterns did not register well either. The actions involving pushing back on Allcare and tightening processes with patients were palatable, particularly if they could blame them on "that managed care company."

Dr. Stuart, Summer Clinic CEO, summarized what he had heard both tonight and as he had worked with Don and his staff on the alternatives, prior to the meeting. "First, we have to lay these concerns out to Allcare very forcefully. They need to know that we are going to push their buttons real hard. Second, related to that, we need to bug the heck out of them. We must do a detailed audit of the funds that they administered and have our actuary review their assumptions on the benefit supplements, in detail. Third, on the medical management side, I support all of Don's recommendations but would add one to it. It's time for a change in the medical director position. Dan is a fine allergist, and he's done yeoman's work in this role for two years now, but it's really beyond his skill set now. I'm proposing that we ask Dr. Sally Cantrell to take the saddle, and that we allocate 10 more hours a week to the job. Those actions are warranted, in my opinion, and can be handled in fairly quick order. I just don't think they are going to be enough. Your thoughts?"

"What I didn't hear anything about was our own administrative capabilities within the MSO," Dr. John Short remarked. "Don and his team are still fairly new to all this, particularly given the product introductions that Allcare has been emphasizing more recently. The number of benefit plans has swelled. Point-of-service is great for the patients, but it's a headache for us. Have you talked to Dan or Deirdre about how they attempt to track those referrals? It's unbelievable! The complexity that we're adding there, often manually, is really hurting our overhead costs. My point is that it's easy to blame Allcare for everything, and they deserve plenty of that, but we also have to look at ourselves and where we are. Our systems need to be much better, to administer this thing."

"Jeff, I'd propose that we leave it at the most basic level of change and see how it works out. We got into this venture to create something different, both for our patients and ourselves. I have the feeling that we're about to create more HMO mechanisms, just like the ones that we deride ourselves. If that's our approach to the business, then why don't we just turn it all back to Allcare? Also, I'm not sure about the change with Dan as medical director. He's a smart guy, a good guy. We've invested in him. He's been attending courses. Besides, I'm not sure how well his allergy practice will come back to support him. Let's not push too far and then regret it." Dr. John Salter, a 52-year-old pediatrician, contributed his conciliatory thoughts.

"John, I don't agree," retorted Dr. Jamie Quinn, a close family practice colleague of Dr. Stuart's. "We need to do all of these things that Don laid out for us. If we go halfway, we're going to find ourselves in even more trouble. I'd suggest that we set a game plan that includes them all; we'll just prioritize the top ones and be realistic about what it takes to implement them. But let's be nothing less than aggressive about this. It's our livelihoods at stake here. More than that, the future of Summer Clinic as a viable group is at stake too."

Two hours later, the Summer Clinic concluded the discussion of its plans to turn around its Allcare commercial capitation contract. Clear direction was provided to Don and his team on a handful of issues, for immediate action. A second set of issues was thornier, though, and required additional discussion and a presentation to the entire partnership, two weeks hence. Finally, some key information was still missing in order to prioritize related actions and to strengthen Summer Clinic's position. Don and his team were asked to obtain that information and come back to the Executive Committee again within two weeks.

ACTION AND RESULTS

After six months, Summer Clinic had fully or partially implemented 60 percent of its turnaround plan. Under less pressing circumstances and less assertive leadership, Summer Clinic would still be debating major action items. Instead, it acted in relative concert to improve its financial performance under capitation. The following actions took place:

1. After a series of sharp exchanges and posturing, Allcare revisited the net premium amounts that it used to calculate Summer's percentage-of-premium capitation. Summer's capitation increased by \$1.30 in total, through monthly increments.

2. Summer Clinic, through an audit, identified $340,000 of payments owed to it by Allcare due to erroneous enrollment and fund administration. Controls were implemented to minimize such discrepancies going forward.
3. Allcare revised its procedures for payment to Summer for care rendered to ineligible members. Additionally, it reduced the period for retroactive disenrollment from six to four months. Combined, these actions reduced Summer's financial exposure on direct, variable health care expenses to $130,000 annually.
4. Dr. Dan Dewitt was replaced, reluctantly after additional debate, as medical director. Dr. Sally Cantrell replaced him in this important role.
5. Internal referral processes, which had been lenient, were expanded and tightened. The Resource Utilization Committee was reconstituted, drawing in three more specialists. Rotation was also established to increase the exposure of more physicians, inside both the group and the IPA, to the utilization management process. Case studies were developed for discussion and education related to challenging utilization and coverage issues. Allcare's health management processes were more effectively integrated into Summer Clinic's Resource Utilization processes to improve communication and clarify benefit interpretation on a real-time basis. Commercial inpatient utilization dropped 10 percent to 215 days per thousand. Specialty referral rates dropped by 15 percent.
6. Working with Allcare, Emergency Room copays were modified to further discourage walk-in utilization. Adjustments were made in Summer Clinic's three urgent care centers to accommodate patients. A promotional campaign related to after-hours care was developed with costs split between Allcare and Summer Clinic on a 50/50 basis. Emergency room visits per thousand dropped 12 percent. Urgent care visits increased 18 percent.
7. Summer Clinic debated its essentially exclusive use of Southside Medical Center. A small contingent of the newer physicians favored moving business incrementally to Northside. They believed strongly that Southside had been arrogant and foolish in not working out a three-way venture with Summer and Allcare early on. Older, established specialists, though, who provided most of the inpatient care, balked. Don Cheek and Dr. Jeff Stuart used the "noise" about a shift

to confront Southside's administration. After two awkward, "finger-pointing" meetings, compromise was reached. Southside Medical Center was brought in on utilization savings with a 1/3 share of the budget. The budget, though, was set at $2.30 pmpm lower than it would have been had Southside entered into a multiyear risk-sharing arrangement two years earlier. Per diems applied against the budget were lowered by 10 percent initially, with additional pricing incentives, based on utilization targets. The likelihood of Southside achieving material financial benefits going forward, though, was severely limited. At the same time, it did maintain its historic relationship with Summer. To maintain some separation, Olney IPA admissions were to be directed incrementally to Southside.

8. A hospital intensivist team was established jointly by the medical center and two Summer Clinic internists to follow closely all acute patients. Hospital-based physicians, specifically in Anesthesia, Radiology, and Neonatology, were encouraged to renegotiate their professional agreements. Incentive programs were established for the hospital-based physicians (HBP) to encourage process improvement. HBP costs dropped by $0.80 pmpm to $6.20 pmpm, still above identified benchmarks.

9. Two specialty agreements covering Ob/Gyn and Oncology were renegotiated under "pseudo-cap" arrangements, narrowing the specialty network modestly to effectuate more patient channeling. Summer, in both cases, chose to work with specialty groups with which it had the longest standing relationships, forgoing more attractive economic options. Two other targeted specialty areas proved to be too complex at the time, with too little clear potential for cost improvement to warrant pursuing.

10. Prescription costs, exploding at double-digit rates of increase, proved to be more problematic. Reluctantly, in return for previous concessions by Allcare, Summer agreed to participate in a shared-risk program for drug costs with risk corridors established and selected applications carved out of the risk. A Pharmacy and Therapeutics Committee was resurrected and reinvigorated. Allcare assigned a Clinical Pharmacologist to work with the Summer physicians. The thorniest issues surrounding Summer's two center pharmacies were resolved through phase-in compromises to be implemented over a one-year period. Prescription drug costs were continuing to escalate

at double-digit rates, but some modest changes in prescribing patterns had been identified and were being reinforced.

11. Summer Clinic, consistent with its desire to be on the "cutting edge" also decided to implement Contact Capitation, a new approach to specialty capitation. Ophthalmology, Urology, and Neurology were selected as "trials" for Contact Cap, with evaluation to occur after 6 and 12 months. Profiling the results within these specialties would be beneficial in determining which specialists were more proficient in a capitated environment. Referrals of Allcare members to those specialists would then be more likely. No results were yet available as the contact cap system was just being implemented.

12. No changes were made in the internal physician compensation system at that time. It had been changed three years prior, and Dr. Jeff Stuart and the other Executive Committee members wanted their full focus on the other changes being implemented internally. Nonetheless, they did appoint a small exploratory compensation committee to review the status of other physician pay systems where substantial capitated care was provided.

13. After much discussion and debate, primary care physician panels were not closed. Allcare successfully urged Summer to make other adjustments to create capacity and to take pressure off its most popular physicians. Two physicians shifted sites to higher growth areas. Two physician assistants were hired and placed under the supervision of the busiest primary care physicians. Finally, appointment hours were shifted modestly and the appointment system was "tweaked" to minimize several inefficiencies that had developed. Even with these changes, Summer Clinic informed Allcare that it would be routinely evaluating its capacity and physician satisfaction under these new arrangements and that panel closures were still a possibility.

14. The fate of Olney IPA proved to be more vexing than expected. As analysis was completed and Summer Clinic MSO staff became more familiar with the operations and network of the IPA, their misgivings about the merger became more pronounced. Their "due diligence" prior to the merger had been so rudimentary that they had not uncovered many of the inadequacies of the IPA. Claims were "discovered." Referral logs were reconciled. Panel enrollment was restated. In short, Summer staff found that they had inherited more

problems to address in the short term, on top of their own capitation challenges. Some of the most intense discussions ensued, amidst a lot of finger pointing, both within Summer and toward the IPA. The Olney physician leaders responded with their own accusations. Ultimately, Summer decided to exercise its option to dissolve the IPA and subcapitate a component of the network. Nonetheless, it took five months of increasing losses before it even got to that decision point and another three months before the subcapitated network was in place as an alternative to the IPA.

15. On the administrative side, Summer, one year after its initial deliberations, transitioned its MSO functions to a nationally recognized company focused on providing services to physician groups at risk. North American Physician Associates (NAPA) agreed to offer an enhanced level of service, commensurate with Allcare's growing product complexity, for a pmpm fee that was 15 percent below what Summer projected their administrative MSO costs to be. Most of the administrative staff in the MSO was assumed by NAPA, easing the transition. Deirdre Pace, though, was replaced with a far more experienced MSO Director.

EPILOGUE—A TURNAROUND

Summer Clinic and its IPA turned around its financial performance under commercial capitation. After one year, the medical group had improved its overall results by 18 percent and trends were favorable or neutral. Allcare membership was growing again with Summer receiving 40,000 of its members. Patient satisfaction was relatively high. Physician turnover was reduced, but some unease still existed. Medical management had grown much more sophisticated. Medicare and Medicaid participation was being carefully analyzed and debated. The next year, Allcare's commercial membership with Summer Clinic reached 45,000 members and financial performance improved another 10 percent.

From a business perspective, Summer Clinic achieved its objective to substantially improve its financial performance under the commercial capitation arrangement with Allcare. It turned around a challenging financial picture. At the same time, though, it found itself evolving more and more as a quasi-insurer, always mindful of risk and business processes. New accountability within the Clinic existed that extended well beyond clinical skills to economic performance. In short, Summer Clinic reflected a business organization with a culture markedly different than its founding and long-time specialist partners would have ever imagined.

SUGGESTED READINGS

Bodenheimer, T. 1999. The American Health Care System—Physicians and the Changing Medical Marketplace. *The New England Journal of Medicine* 304, No. 7.

Boland, P. 1993. *Making Managed Healthcare Work.* Gaithersburg, MD: Aspen Publishers, Inc.

Goldstein, D. 1995. Easing the Transition to Capitation. *MedNews* XI, No. 1: 4–5.

Goldstein, D. 1996. Building and Managing Effective Physicians Organizations. *Marketing Dynamics, American Medical News.*

Grumbach, K. et al. 1998. Primary Care Physicians' Experience of Financial Incentives in Managed-Care Systems. *The New England Journal of Medicine* 339, No. 21.

Health plan strives to create true partnership with capitated physicians. 1999. *Capitation Management Report* 6, No. 2: 25–28.

Iezzoni, L. and Ayanian, J. 1998. Paying More Fairly for Medicare Capitated Care. *The New England Journal of Medicine* 339, No. 26.

Kao, A. et al. 1998. The Relationship between Method of Physician Payment and Patient Trust. *The Journal of the American Medical Association* 280: 1708–1714.

Kongstvedt, P. 1989. *The Managed Health Care Handbook.* Rockville, MD: Aspen Publishers, Inc.

Kuttner, R. 1998. The Risk-Adjustment Debate. *The New England Journal of Medicine* 339, No. 26.

CHAPTER 3

Power to the Specialists through Contract Capitation

Clifford R. Frank, MHSA, and Timothy M. Davlantes, MD

The tension in the room grew as the IPA President, Dr. Hamilton, quietly approached the podium. More than 50 physician leaders from area hospitals were gathered to hear the latest physician response to managed care encroachment on physician incomes and clinical decision making.

Dr. Hamilton looked about the room and waited patiently for quiet. At the appropriate moment he began to make his case as to why physicians should accept the mantle of global capitation in managed care contracting.

"This is the last trench in our fight with managed care. Global capitation is the way we get back our power over clinical decisions, the way we stabilize our incomes, and the way we maintain our patient base. We've seen the corrosive impact of managed care on our professional lives as the paperwork headaches and hassles grow each month, while our fees are cut. We've seen the payers play one doctor against another, one group against another, and one hospital against another. We've seen the arrival of practice management companies determined to siphon off lucrative hospital services into Wall Street's pockets with the complicity of managed care payers. Physician-driven global capitation can change the end of this story. But if we don't fight here, if we don't fight now, our last trench will be overrun and nothing will be left but surrender to the insurance company chieftains."

The call to the barricades was only the beginning. Many difficult decisions confronted the IPA leadership as they sought to build a sustainable organization capable of managing global capitation contracts. In many ways the market had made their job of selling the concept easier, but the job of delivering positive results more difficult. The payers had already harvested the easy savings. Payers in this southeastern community had already lowered fee schedules to 100 percent of Medicare or less for specialists. Primary care was still capitated, but their capitation rates were under pressure as well. Payers had also narrowed panels by terminating "high utilizing" or "uncooperative" physicians. Some payers had implemented single specialty capitation programs in several specialties such as mental health, cardiology, ENT, orthopedics, and others. These efforts by payers had resulted in network inpatient utilization declines to 250 days/1,000 commercial HMO and 1,340 days/1,000 Medicare HMO.

Dr. Hamilton continued, "Our challenge today is to bring our physicians and hospitals together to present not a wall, but a better path for payers to take. If we can show managed care payers how much more we physicians can save them, we can share in the savings of our own efforts. Today, every time you avoid a procedure or discharge a patient, you're saving somebody else money. Under global capitation, those savings are yours."

Questions from physician leaders began almost before Dr. Hamilton had finished his opening remarks. "What makes you think we can do this better than the insurance companies?" asked one. "Why should we trust the hospital this time?" asked another. "Who is going to determine who gets the capitation?" worried a third.

"The insurers are big, and distant, and they're not doctors. They know how to manage price. They don't know anything about managing care. We do. We've just never been paid to do it, but under global capitation we'll make more money by managing the care. Insurers are good at pitting us against each other, but we're the ones making decisions about patient care. We're the ones spending the money. We're the ones who can save it too. Under global capitation, we have both the ability and the reason to go the extra mile for the patient to avoid a more costly expense," Dr. Hamilton intoned.

"The hospital is full of waste. How many times have you been ready to discharge a patient at 7 PM. and been told to hold the patient until the hospital discharge staff is there in the morning? How many times have you been told you can't get a test on the weekend when you could otherwise send the patient home? How much bureaucracy and paper shuffling have you had to endure to get something you need from the hospital? What clout do we have with the hospital now? Not much individually. But, under global capitation, what we do affects the hospital and how much they get paid. We don't have to pay for a patient who gets parked in the hospital because their processes don't work," Dr. Hamilton said to rising physician interest.

"The hospital needs physician allies in their fights with managed care. They need us to help save them money on their contracts, and we need them to not contract with every jackleg HMO. Together we can help the good payers do better, and make the bad payers suffer." Some heads started nodding in agreement.

Dr. Hamilton continued, "The IPA is currently open to all medical staff of the health system, but that will end soon. The IPA is inclusive. It is designed to embrace our medical staff, not carve it up. But a time will come when we only need X many of this specialty, and additional applications may not be considered. Our intent is to go to plans and say, 'This is our physician panel. These are the doctors who will perform under global capitation.' If a payer has a problem with somebody on the panel, we will deal with that on a case-by-case basis. This is an inclusive IPA. We want your involvement and we want your voice to be heard."

The room exploded in applause and the IPA was launched.

CAPITATION CONTEXT

Capitation as a payment method has not always worked to the advantage of the providers of care. In the IPA's market, capitated single specialty networks have been present for seven years. These specialty networks receive a product-specific capitation payment from the HMOs and pay physicians either on a fee schedule with a withhold, or on a floating fee schedule that balances to the funds available in the pool each month. In either case, the fundamental incentives facing physicians have not changed— more services equal more money. These specialty networks have had to reduce their payment levels to physicians over time, as the flaws in the payment system became evident to the participants. In addition, medical management has become more intrusive, even among the physician-driven single specialty networks. Because the networks are using fee-for-service payments in one form or another, the incentives facing individual physicians are to encourage, not discourage unnecessary utilization.

Another unanticipated market dynamic of single specialty capitation has been the increased ability of payers to swap specialty networks in order to obtain a lower per member per month rate. Every three years or more often, payers have bid out specialty services in ophthalmology, ENT, cardiology, gastroenterology, mental health, and others in an effort to drive price lower. The effect has been dramatic with per member per month prices falling 20–30 percent. In addition, payers have unilaterally imposed price cuts on specialty networks in mid-contract without so much as a negotiation. Single specialty network capitation makes implementing such changes easier for payers as they have only one dollar figure to evaluate because they have shifted the utilization risk onto the network.

Network hopping by payers adversely affects physicians, patients, and employers. However, network hopping can improve a payer's selection of risk by inducing sick members to stay with their cardiologist while the network switches specialty panels. PCPs lose track as to which specialists are eligible to receive their referrals, and they lose control as to whom they can refer. Patients get aggravated at the splintering of care, particularly if the various specialists they seek are geographically distant from their PCP or other specialists they see.

More recently, payers have started adding outpatient facility costs to single specialty capitation programs such as ophthalmology and ENT. In these situations, payers are incentivising physicians to seek lower cost facilities on their own, which may either mean special price concessions from hospitals or using freestanding facilities in lieu of higher priced hospital-based services. Physicians see these arrangements as opportunities to obtain facility savings dollars at the expense of their local community hospital.

While IPAs have been forming and negotiating their entry into global capitation, the specialty fee-for-service world has not remained stable. Many HMOs and PPOs have first moved to Medicare-based fee schedules resulting in substantial cuts in payments to specialists. Then, these same payers have reduced the conversion factors thereby further reducing historical payment levels. As payers feel pricing pressure from increases in prescription drug costs and technology enhancements, they have resorted to further fee schedule reductions. The cuts usually are across the board; not targeted cuts aimed at particular high-utilizing specialties or specialists. The use of this blunt instrument has resulted in inequities of pain in that efficient physicians are enjoying the same whack as inefficient ones. The efficient individual physician is routinely sacrificed on the mantle of payer system limitations.

The political issues facing Dr. Hamilton in the formation of an IPA were complex and interwoven with historical physician/hospital issues that have complicated medical politics for many years. The IPA leadership knew that payers would continue to pursue a divide and conquer strategy where possible. By forming a partnership with the health system, the IPA hoped to be able to generate enough counterforce in the market so as to induce the HMOs to negotiate at-risk contracts that would return savings to physicians from improvements in the clinical efficiencies they created. For that strategy to work, however, providers had to either offer a compelling vision, and/or have the ability to say "no" to a substandard contract offer from a payer.

Dr. Hamilton soon learned that providers are loath to walk away from a revenue stream. Around the meeting table such devotion to a revenue source, no matter how bad, became known as "green cocaine." The physicians' addiction to an in-place revenue stream made the payers' leverage much greater in dealings across the negotiation table. Individual physicians could not withstand the potential disruption of even a relatively small amount of patient revenue. The result has been a series of unilateral fee cuts by payers, and their unwillingness to globally capitate unless required to do so by market forces.

Another more insidious disruption Dr. Hamilton encountered occurred when dealing with hospital-based physicians: radiology, pathology, anesthesiology, and emergency. These physicians were reluctant to move away from their high historical payment levels. As a result, payers paid less to other physician specialties. And in looking at capitation, these hospital-based specialists were understandably concerned that they had little control over utilization of services within their specialty. Dr. Hamilton and the IPA faced difficulty in convincing these specialists that their livelihood was tied to the livelihood of their referral sources. In more than one case the hospitals hosting these specialists became involved with discussions up to and including threats to terminate their exclusive hospital contracts if these specialists did not participate with the IPA on the same basis as other physicians. It was not a happy situation for any party.

Physician leaders began to understand the imperative driving the IPA and the health system in their collaborative efforts—to regain control of the medical management process and harvest the savings from improving clinical efficiency. Such vision, while shared at the leadership level, was difficult to disseminate to individual physicians scattered about the community. Such vision was quickly forgotten as financial pressures on the IPA mounted. Such vision was briefly recaptured when annual bonuses were distributed, but soon again forgotten as employer premium pressures eliminated the possibility of raising physician payment levels.

THE IPA IS BORN

Out of the turmoil and change that was occurring in the market, the IPA was born. The IPA was formed by a core group of physicians with a common vision. One core principle was the concept of "inclusivity with loyalty." The basic premise was that all physicians should be given the opportunity to participate in the IPA once their loyalty to the organization and its partner, Health System, was established. To determine "loyalty" the physician members needed to meet two tests. First, the physician needed to have active staff privileges at one of the Health System facilities. Second, the physician's admitting activity was verified by reviewing public information discharge data by the hospital to determine that greater that 50 percent of the physician's practice was in fact situated at a Health System facility.

Another core principle of the IPA founders was that decisions would be data driven. As part of this premise, all physicians agreed to supply data on their practice to the IPA. Specifically, specialists were compelled to release data on their practice to the primary care physicians. This was met with some resistance by some of the specialists, and ultimately, some decided not to participate.

The third core principle was that the IPA be physician driven. The founders of the IPA realized that physicians needed to be in the senior leadership roles of the IPA. Physicians bring a unique perspective to organizational management that is often not present in non-physician managers. As a result, the IPA decided that the President and CEO must be a physician.

Another core principle proved to be one of the most debated issues in the formation of the IPA. The IPA founders, most of whom were specialists, recognized that the success of the organization would require a majority representation of PCPs on the IPA Board of Directors. The local market had been littered with the remains of failed specialist-dominated managed care organizations. The local Medical Society had a specialist-dominated plan that failed, and two local hospitals had specialist-dominated partnerships with HMOs that also had failed.

The decision to create a majority of Board seats for PCPs was further complicated by the fact that the Health System had employed a number of PCPs. Some physicians were concerned that allocating a majority of Board seats to PCPs would allow the Health System to gain control of the IPA. Describing the nature of the PCP seats on the Board mitigated this concern.

It was decided that employed PCPs should not dominate the PCP Board seats.

Another core principle was that the physicians would share equally in any gains or losses realized by the IPA. This concept of "shared pain, shared gain" helped allay the fears of some physicians who were concerned their efforts might be thwarted by the actions of others.

Another principle that is core to the organization is the insistence of full delegation from the payer. Full delegation includes the ability to make medical management and credentialing decisions. Furthermore, provider servicing would be a required activity of the IPA. Physicians wanted to avoid having multiple office audits and reviews by multiple HMOs, in favor of their own organization performing those obligatory reviews to maintain compliance with the various accrediting agencies. Finally, the IPA insisted on full claims delegation. The claim represents the core standardized data element in medical practice. The organization that controls the data is best positioned to control their destiny. The IPA did not want to be subject to the vagaries of payer claims processing. Also, timely, efficient, and fair reimbursement was key to obtaining early physician commitment to the IPA.

The final core principle on which the IPA was founded was the idea of specialty accountability through specialty-specific budgets. Each specialty was allocated a specific monthly budget for physician services. The specialty budget was not shared with physicians in other specialties. This preserved the autonomy of the specialists while preventing the depletion of their specialty pool by the actions of a non-affiliated specialty. The orthopedic surgeons were not affected by the actions of the general surgeons or the oncologists.

THE IPA TAKES CONTROL

With the principles in place and the organization established, the IPA was now ready to take back control of medical decision making from the HMOs. The key to achieving this was to accept the financial responsibility for those clinical decisions. The IPA knew they needed to build a medical management infrastructure to manage the financial risk. The first step was to identify a medical director to lead the development effort. The early medical management processes revolved around existing hospital-based activities. A precertification unit was established and basic medical management protocols were instituted. Concurrent review and case management activities were instituted, and the IPA was ready to pursue contracts with HMOs.

In early negotiations with payers, the IPA used its partnership with the hospitals to exert additional market clout. The alignment with the hospitals afforded the IPA access to capital as well as physical space and telecommunications and information services infrastructure. Incentives were created to encourage payers to contract with Maxim Health. Payers that contracted with Maxim Health were given favored hospital rates, where those that chose not to contract with Maxim Health were either not offered hospital contracts at all or were given less favorable rates.

Then, in early 1996, the first contract was signed. A "pilot" program was instituted for the management of approximately 3,500 HMO lives. The IPA now had a chance to show that they could deliver on the promise of decreased cost while maintaining quality. Would the principles defined at the formation of the IPA sustain the organization? Would the physicians keep focused on the common goal, or would individualism take over? Would the negotiated percent of premium be enough to meet the utilization demand? Over the next few months the IPA would learn the answers to these questions and face other unanticipated challenges.

IMPLEMENTING THE FIRST CONTRACT

At the outset, the IPA had established separate budgeted specialty pools. Now the challenge was how to distribute the pools each month to all the specialists within each pool. Primary care services were paid under prospective capitation and thus initially did not expose the IPA to the risk of overpayment of the pool. Specialty care payments, however, were initially established on a fee-for-service basis. The concern here was that the potential existed for the pool to be overspent if utilization of specialty services exceeded the projected budgetary allocation.

The IPA leadership recognized that the fee-for-service payment methodology served as a transitional model until an acceptable capitation model could be developed. Initially fee-for-service reimbursement was tied to 100 percent of Medicare allowable, with a 50 percent withhold. The fact that the physicians supported this indicated the level of commitment that was present at the start of the IPA. The 50 percent withhold was necessary to protect the organization from unexpected expenses from any specialty.

After two months, it was evident that the experience of this small group did not require a 50 percent withhold, and it was reduced to 10 percent. However, the risk of overspending the specialty pools still existed.

MANAGING THE RISK OF GLOBAL CAPITATION

The hardest thing for an IPA to do is to reduce payments to its physicians. Using a fee schedule to pay physicians is simple, sounds safe, and within the context of capitation usually results in disaster. Like a gambler looking for the next hand to get back to even, IPA Boards are reluctant to cut fees in the hope of having a next good month. The result is that tough decisions get postponed, and the monthly deficits grow larger. IPA was no exception to this IPA management dynamic. The fee-for-service with a 10 percent withhold worked during the early months, but was doomed as winter's sicker months loomed ahead. At the end of the first nine months some specialties were in surplus, and some were in deficit. The IPA was supposed to reduce payments to those that were in deficit so that each specialty bore their own burdens.

However, the IPA Board realized such steps would be divisive and make difficult sustaining physician support for the nascent IPA. In some specialties, the experience on 3,500 lives just was not statistically reliable to result in fee cuts. For example, in oncology there were six cases instead of three, but there was little physician discretion in the utilization of physician resources involved. Adjusting the oncologists' payments would penalize them for the epidemiological risk over which they had no control. Some members of the IPA Board thought such an adjustment was appropriate because they were in the insurance business through risk contracts. Others felt that the oncologists should bear the discretionary professional services utilization risk, but not the epidemiological risk of cancer occurrences.

Another problem with the fee-for-service with withhold payment method was that aggressive utilization by one specialist adversely affected other specialists within the specialty pool. This unhappy circumstance was highlighted among gynecologists who had wildly differing practice patterns. The same situation existed in ophthalmology. The inequity of paying physicians fee-for-service out of a capitated pool and then asking them to be prudent in their utilization was proving to be unrealistic. Each month, the conservative doctors were paid less, and the aggressive proceduralists received more from the specialty pool. The IPA Board worried about the utilization behavior such a fee-for-service payment method rewarded.

The IPA Board had also received considerable feedback from the physician membership that primary care physicians were continuing to closely regulate specialty physician delivery of care. Referrals were often for evaluation only. Treatment referrals were for one to three visits requiring a callback to the PCP for approval of additional visits. Such visits usually were approved, but the process was burdensome to all parties including the IPA, which had to administer the cumbersome referral authorization process. Specialists reminded Board members that the goals of the IPA were to simplify care processes, not add a new level of burden. Specialists also chafed at the idea that they were at risk for the cost of specialty services, but not allowed to perform their specialty without undue hassle from PCPs, the IPA, or the Plan. One PCP Board member suggested that the PCPs were really doing the specialists a favor by overseeing their specialty colleagues' care to prevent unnecessary utilization. The specialists in the room scoffed at the PCP's assertion of the PCP's protective value to at-risk specialists. They felt that PCPs routinely approve things that perhaps they should not, and specialists observed that PCPs object to things that routinely made good sense to specialists. Moreover, several specialists pointed out that PCPs were in fact more likely to turf a case to capitated specialists so as to lighten their own patient load. All this tension between primary care and specialty physicians was destructive to the IPA and disruptive to patient care.

THE MOVE TO CONTACT CAPITATION

At the quarterly IPA Board meeting, Dr. Hamilton rose to explain the dilemma facing IPA physicians. "Ladies and gentlemen, what we have here is about to become a colossal mess unless we fix it now. We have 3,500 lives now, with 25,000 more coming in three months. We've had some specialties come in under their budgets, and others that are well over. But fundamentally, we haven't changed anything yet. We have doctors still paid fee-for-service, albeit against a specialty pool, but the incentives the individual practitioner faces are still the same as under fee-for-service. This is destined to fail. This system is dysfunctional, and we have to change it."

The IPA Board members grew edgy even though many of these payment issues had been worked through the IPA committee structure. They knew that the time was approaching for a new payment method, and they were all nervous about it. Contact Capitation. They knew the term, but found the whole formulation so different than the fee schedule payment methods of other plans.

Dr. Hamilton continued, "What we are here to discuss today is a payment system called contact capitation. Contact capitation is a method used in many West Coast IPAs and other organizations to divvy up a specialty pool. The way it works generally is this: Each physician in a given specialty turns in his or her claims as he or she does today. But instead of receiving payment for each service, the physician receives payment for each patient he or she is managing. Each patient you see gets on your list and stays on your list for a year. At the end of each month we figure out how many patients are being managed within the specialty and how many patients are on each physician's list. You get your pro rata share of the specialty pool based on how many patients are on your list. If you have 7 percent of the patients, you get 7 percent of the specialty pool."

The questions started immediately. "If I see a patient six times or one time, I get the same money?" asked a general surgeon.

"Yes," replied Dr. Hamilton. "Under contact capitation we're counting patients, not procedures. Now we know that sometimes you'll see a patient just for a consult, but most of the time you're seeing them for more than that. Your responsibility is to manage the care for that patient in your specialty for 12 consecutive months, and you will get paid for that patient each of those 12 months."

The general surgeon followed up with a sharp attack. "You mean to tell me that a gall bladder and a colon resection patient count the same?"

Dr. Hamilton reflected a moment and said, "In a way, yes. All patients count the same unless a specialty wants to make adjustments for certain kinds of patients within their specialty. For example, I'm an oncologist. We probably would count leukemia patients greater than we would a standard oncology patients because of the time and intensity of resources that leukemia patients require."

A gastroenterology physician intervened, "Are you saying that each specialty makes those decisions about fairness issues? We have some people in our specialty that do certain procedures such as an Endoscopic Retro Cholangeal Pyelogram (ERCP) that others do not. Those people doing ERCPs would get hurt in this system unless there was some sort of adjustment."

"That's what I'm saying," sighed Dr. Hamilton. "Each specialty knows best what can throw a system like this out of whack. It's up to them to determine weights and carve-outs and other adjustments to make it fair to the specialists involved. We have lead physicians in each specialty that will convene a meeting of five to six specialists to go over the details of this model and identify the adjustment factors their specialty wants to use. We'll load those factors into the computer system and apply them to the contact points each month to make the system fair."

Dr. Hamilton sensed an open moment and he pounced, "Contact capitation allows specialty physicians to take responsibility for the care of their patients without the imposition of clinical value systems that we may not agree with. With contact capitation, the referral from the PCP lasts 12 months. The phone tag and hassle for more visits is gone because it is up to you, the specialist, as to how you want to treat the patient. Of course if you're going to perform a procedure that is costly, it will still need to be precertified through the utilization management function, but that is now to your advantage. Remember, you're not getting paid more to do more. You're getting paid to manage a population of patients in your specialty. It is your responsibility to do it cost effectively, and if you don't, you waste your time—not your colleagues' money."

A gynecologist on the IPA Board perked up at that idea. The gynecologists had been having a great deal of trouble with the diversity of practice patterns within their specialty. The result was that some practitioners were performing services far more often than their colleagues, and their practice patterns had created a sizeable deficit in the gynecology specialty capitation pool. The fee-for-service payments to these aggressive gynecologists were coming at the expense of the other gynecologists in the pool, and it was causing substantial tensions as doctors began to realize how a few aggressive physicians could bankrupt a capitation pool.

The gynecologist asked, "You mean that if I'm treating 40 patients, and Dr. So-and-so is treating 40 patients, but he is operating on twice as many patient as I am, we get the same money?"

"Yes, that's right," said Dr. Hamilton. "With contact capitation, you are no longer at risk for your colleagues' unfavorable practice patterns. They bear that cost directly. Now they may not be too happy with this, but we'll give them the data so they can see where they are different than their specialty colleagues, and they'll be motivated to address the problem, unlike today."

The primary care physicians on the IPA Board had been quiet to this point. But now one senior practitioner rose to object to the methodology. "I am disturbed at the quality aspects of physicians being paid the same whether they perform a procedure or not. Seems to me that the risk of undertreatment might be significant."

Dr. Hamilton almost lost his temper. Primary care physicians in the IPA had squeezed the Board for higher primary care capitation rates, and now this primary care physician was worrying about specialists locking their doors to enhance their payment levels. Dr. Hamilton icily replied, "Well, Phil, it hasn't bothered you being a capitated primary care physician, has it? Look, with contact capitation, doctors don't get paid unless they see patients. If a specialist drags the care or turfs the case, the primary care doctors are going to get upset and redirect referrals away from those specialists. The primary care physicians are the key to quality assurance. If you're not happy with the care a specialist is giving your patients, refer the patients to somebody else. If a patient starts seeing another specialist, the contact capitation payment to the first specialist stops when the payment to the second specialist starts. And the second specialist gets a full 12 months' contact payment, because we want to make sure he or she is well taken care of and that he or she will take good care of the patient. The primary care physicians still have a major role in guiding the care process. Contact capitation doesn't take that away. Contact capitation takes away the daily grind of limited referrals and requests from specialists for more visits."

The primary care physician resumed his seat. The question was called, and the vote taken. The resolution to institute contact capitation moved forward. Next was the implementation phase.

SINGLE SPECIALTY CAPITATION RATE DEVELOPMENT

Key to contact capitation is the development of single specialty budgets. These budgets are usually product specific, such as for Medicare, Medicaid, and commercial HMO populations. An important part of the specialty budget development is ascertaining the overlaps between specialties and making sure that the money and the work end up properly reflected in the same actuarial bucket. For example, in this community the gastroenterologists usually perform colonoscopies. However, in the actuarial data on which the specialty pools were built colonoscopies were assigned to the colon-rectal surgeons. This resulted in overpayments to the colon-rectal surgeons and underfunding of the gastroenterology pool. The inequity was discovered by looking at the fee-for-service equivalent yield for the colon-rectal surgeons. After reviewing the data, the IPA moved $.15 pmpm from the colon-rectal pool to the gastroenterology pool. The money stays with the work. The IPA was determined there should be no substantial windfalls due to actuarial allocation deviations.

Occasionally these specialty budgets can also be stratified by age depending upon the delivery system configuration. In the case of Maxim Health, pediatric specialty services were primarily delivered by pediatric specialists within one multispecialty clinic. Creating separate pediatric and adult pools resulted in less confusion among the physicians treating just adult patients.

However, the creation of separate pediatric and adult pools also highlighted the problem of overlaps between adult physicians who treat children and the pediatric specialty clinic. These situations occurred mostly in ENT, ophthalmology, and dermatology. In addressing the situation, the IPA faced two important questions: Should all pediatric specialty care be directed to the specialty clinic, and how could the pediatric specialty clinic be compensated for its presumed more severe case mix?

In looking at whether the pediatric specialty clinic should capture all pediatric specialty care within the community, the IPA's value of inclusiveness rose to the surface. The debate focused on the perception that the pediatric specialty clinic provided higher quality of care juxtaposed against the IPA's need to include these community physicians in the network. Those community physicians made their feelings known about being potentially restricted to adult medicine only. They sent a delegation to an IPA Board meeting to let the Board know that such a restriction would eliminate the IPA's adult network in those specialties as they were not about to surrender about one-third of their patients to the children's clinic.

Once that issue was resolved in favor of including community physicians for pediatric care, the issue of severity adjustment became critical to retaining the pediatric specialty clinic in the network. They argued that they handle a large number of congenital situations, retreatments of other's care, and esoteric referrals from the community physicians. If their payments were not severity adjusted, the clinic could not participate on the same basis as other specialty physicians.

At the urging of the IPA leadership, the interested parties convened a meeting to come to some accommodation. Administrators explained how contact capitation works and how cases could be weighted for severity, complexity, or other factors. The pediatric specialty clinic representatives argued that not all their cases were more severe, but on average there was a substantial difference. The community physicians agreed that on average the pediatric specialty clinic did indeed see sicker patients including ones in their specialties of dermatology, ophthalmology, and ENT. The group worked on developing a set of distinguishing diagnoses that could be given supplemental contact weights to adjust for the resources such diagnoses required. However, the discussions soon bogged down on esoteric clinical disputes. Finally, the administrator of the pediatric specialty clinic suggested a breakthrough alternative. He suggested using a provider-based weight that would weight the pediatric specialty clinic contacts overall, not diagnosis- or procedure-specific. Such an overall weight would have the effect of raising the pediatric specialty clinic's average payment per contact without unduly burdening the administrative process with additional complications. The community physicians suggested a supplemental severity weight of 20 percent meaning that the pediatric specialty clinic's contacts would count 20 percent more than the community physicians of the same specialty. All parties agreed that such a weight seemed fair, but they would periodically evaluate it to ensure that the supplemental adjustment was warranted.

CONTACT CAPITATION WEIGHTS AND CARVE-OUTS

In the specialty meetings where contact capitation was explained, the fairness refinements necessary to make contact capitation work in each specialty were developed. In gynecology, the specialists decided that gyn/oncology patients should be weighted three times the average gyn patients. That meant that gyn-oncology patients were worth 36 contact points per year instead of 12. In ophthalmology, the retina subspecialists convinced their colleagues that their patients were fundamentally different than general ophthalmology patients. To resolve the issue, the ophthalmologists created a contact capitation subpool for only retina physicians. In cardiology, the physicians created an invasive cardiology subpool because invasive cardiology services were fundamentally different than clinical cardiology patients. The resolution of the problem was to create an invasive cardiology contact capitation subpool using selected procedure codes to define the subpool. Cardiac caths, stents, nuclear cardiology, and other costly diagnostic procedures were included in this invasive cardiology pool, and physicians were paid contact capitation from it. Cardiologists providing clinical cardiology services generated their contact points from a separate clinical cardiology pool. In the case of cardiology, it was possible for a patient to generate both a clinical cardiology contact and an invasive cardiology contact if they received those services as well.

Other specialties made minor adjustments. Local community physicians looking at their specialties made these decisions and determined what they felt was fair. Over time some additional adjustments had to be made as new situations developed. Some urologists perform office chemotherapy. Others do not. To avoid inequities within the specialty, a supplemental contact weight had to be developed for office chemotherapy.

RESULTS ACHIEVED

Payment levels to physicians through contact capitation have remained at market levels while other HMOs not contracting with IPA have lowered their specialist fee schedules. The contact capitation payment system has resulted in variable payments to physicians based upon their individual utilization of services. Some physicians did well with contact capitation, while others did not. In certain specialties, the compression around the mean was strong resulting in fairly common payment levels among physicians of that specialty. In others, the payment levels were quite diverse. For example, in gynecology some physicians' payment levels yielded fee-for-service equivalent payments as low as 50 percent of Medicare while others were as high as 160 percent of Medicare in the same specialty. Some physicians feel these variations in payment are due to differences in case mix and severity. Others in the same specialty feel such differences are the result of differences in practice patterns. Additional studies are underway to determine if special weightings or other adjustments are warranted.

Utilization of hospital services has been within expected levels, but hospital days have not been reduced beyond standard HMO levels. Contact capitation by itself has not been sufficient to alter physician behavior beyond modest changes in patient management. Where the IPA invested in physician education and presentation of relevant data, contact capitation helped to heighten physician interest in and responsiveness to treatment alternatives. However, physicians continue to present constant managerial challenges without end.

Utilization of ancillary services has continued at levels consistent with actuarial expectations, but anecdotal evidence is emerging of steady altering of treatment processes, particularly in the treatment of chronic diseases. In cardiology, the physicians developed their own treatment program for congestive heart failure (CHF) and started a CHF clinic for medication and education.

For emergency room (ER) care, the ER pool was recently combined with the primary care pool and case rates for ER physicians were implemented. These case rates are now charged against the primary care pool, and primary care physicians are most interested in providing alternatives to the emergency room for minor ailments. Several physician offices have moved to extended hours and one primary care group has started an after-hours clinic for capitated patients. In addition, a local pediatric group has started an after-hours program for children that is available until 11 PM. each night.

Utilization of prescription drugs has been higher than expected and has contributed to significant financial pressure within the global capitation arrangement. Prescription drug utilization was budgeted at about $14 pmpm and actual utilization was closer to $20 pmpm. Some of the increase in prescription drug utilization was the result of industry trends in terms of new drugs, new applications for existing patented drugs, and lower than hoped for formulary compliance. But evidence exists for at least four other reasons for increased prescription drug utilization.

First, with contact capitation some cases that could be managed aggressively or conservatively are managed by observing the development of symptoms and testing various therapies, including medications. Surgical intervention may be held back in lieu of alternatives that are less invasive in cases that could reasonably be managed medically or surgically.

Second, in some cases medical management may eliminate the need for procedural intervention, such as in the case of ulcer therapy. We now know that with the right antibiotic therapy, many ulcers can be eliminated without the use of endoscopy. With contact capitation, medical interventions seem to get more serious consideration than when fee schedules are used to pay for additional marginal procedures.

Third, physicians have an interest in making sure they prescribe the full therapeutic drug regimen to enhance the chances of patients making a full recovery from their illnesses. The medical literature is replete with examples of medical interventions that are incomplete and less than fully effective because patients did not receive the full complement of prescription medications relevant to their particular illness or condition. With contact capitation, physicians have an incentive to be more diligent in this area.

Fourth, physicians have an interest in enhancing patient compliance with medication directives. Noncompliant patients result in more physician time spent on the consequences of such noncompliant behavior—time that is not additionally compensated. With contact capitation, physicians have an incentive to reach out to their patients to increase medication regimen compliance and improve their patients' overall health.

Physician office staff have struggled to integrate contact capitation payments into their normal business office routines. Posting capitation payments is well understood by primary care physician offices, but is still a new phenomenon to specialist offices. The explanation of payment and patient roster that accompany the check to each specialist provides enough information for payment posting if staff are trained in its use. Office staff training was underemphasized in the initial rollout of contact capitation. As time has unfolded, these lessons have been learned, but at a cost of a great deal of day-to-day frustration. Physician office staff know how to take write-offs. But contact capitation requires them sometimes to post payments to patient accounts for whom no service was billed that month. When talking to physician office staff, the IPA administrative staff learned not to use the phrase "negative contractual" even though it meant something to the IPA. Such a term just sent physician staff over the edge. Helping them identify ways to set up special write-off codes, and set up dummy charge codes to apply against capitation payments helped solve the office administrative problems.

ADMINISTRATIVE ASPECTS OF CONTACT CAPITATION

The IPA learned quickly that explaining contact capitation was easy compared to the challenge of administering it. Conventional managed care claims systems are not designed to handle episode of care payment methodologies. As a result, several modifications to basic administrative processes were made, including claims flow, pool payout amounts, retroactive adjustments, and contact severity/complexity weighting.

With the implementation of the contact capitation program, claims flow changed. The first issue the IPA had to decide was when a contact began. The physicians argued that a contact began when a patient sees the specialist—the date of service. The IPA administrators argued that a contact began when the claim was received by the IPA—the date of receipt. Both parties presented sound arguments. Using a date-of-service trigger for initiating a contact best fits how physicians think about their patients, particularly those on a recall system. Physicians measure elapsed time between visits such as a six-month recall, an annual exam, or a periodic screening. However, using date-of-service adds administrative complications because claims are not necessarily promptly submitted by physicians. The resulting ebb and flow of claims could result in more variability from month to month of the number of contacts active in any given period.

Using date-of-service as the contact trigger means that the transition process to contact capitation would be cumbersome and stretched out for several months. By using date-of-service as the trigger, claims with earlier dates-of-service would have to be paid fee-for-service, thereby creating two payment processes for a period of time. But, paying the old claims' run out under fee-for-service would allow physicians to maintain their cash flow as the claims were accumulated for contact capitation.

However, using date-of-service also creates a windfall problem. It takes a few months for the contact volume in a specialty to reach its predicted level because old patients are being paid fee-for-service. If the administrators pay out the full specialty capitation in the early months, the value of a patient contact in the early months will be substantially overstated. As the contact volume builds each month, the value of any individual contact would commensurately decline. A contact in Month 1 or Month 2 might be worth $150 and in Month 7 only worth $30. To avoid such perverse outcomes from using a date-of-service contact trigger, the IPA was going to hold back some funds from each specialty pool to payout in later months as the number of new contacts built to the expected level. The IPA's goal was to maintain a fairly stable contact value from month to month so that wild swings in payments would be avoided.

An alternative approach was to use the date-of-receipt of the claim on the patient as the contact trigger mechanism. This method was favored by the IPA administrators because of its simplicity. Because the claims would be all counted the same way from the start of the cutover, no reserving was required for contact build-up. The claims stream would simply be counted in a different manner starting at the cutover date. Claims received after the cutover date (January 1) would be contact capitation claims. Claims received prior to that date would be paid fee-for-service. The physicians were concerned that although their colleagues had agreed to contact capitation, they had so agreed as of a fixed point in time—presumably for patient visits after that time. The IPA's contract amendment read for claims submitted after the cutover date. How could the IPA pay contact capitation for patients with dates-of-service prior to the cutover date?

The IPA chose to use date-of-service for services provided after the cutover date of January 1. For services provided before the cutover date, the IPA would pay based on the old fee schedule.

At the same time as contact capitation was switching on, the IPA's membership grew fivefold resulting in other potential problems—windfalls. The situation developed that at the end of the first month, only the IPA had received a small number of claims for services provided in the first month. To pay contact capitation on those few services would have resulted in physicians receiving 300 to 400 percent of Medicare for those initial contacts. The IPA chose to combine the first and second months into one payment, thereby allowing more time for claims to accumulate. At the end of the second month, more claims from January had arrived. But few claims from February had been received, thereby replicating the problem from the month before. The IPA leadership reviewed the situation and made an administrative decision to limit payment to any physician to no more than 150 percent of Medicare. Each physician's contacts would carry forward, but the payment would be limited to no more than 150 percent of Medicare on a fee-for-service equivalent basis. The result was that in the early months, some money was left in specialty pools each month because of the individual payment ceiling. But by about Month 5, the claims flow had normalized, and contacts were accumulating as expected. This steady claim flow generated enough contacts to bring payment levels per contact well below the ceiling levels, thereby using all the funds in the specialty pools, as expected. The windfall protection intervention did its job of smoothing the contact payment levels throughout the implementation of a large number of new IPA enrollees.

The regularity of the contact flow was important in maintaining a relative stable value of contacts within each specialty. Wide swings in the value of a contact within a specialty were not desirable as such swings create anxiety and suspicion among the physician panel. Stability can be maintained if the flow of contacts is consistent from month to month. However, several factors can disrupt that consistency including seasonality of particularly diseases or conditions, fluctuations in chargebacks to the specialty pool, changes in referral patterns, and changes in IPA enrollment. These fluctuations can be managed through the use of payout ceilings as noted above or reserving funds from less active months to more active months. Such reserving of pool funds can take place at the time the pool funds are created each month. If contact volume is down, funds can be carried over until contact volume picks up. If contact volume is greater than expected, the value of any individual contact will decline until contact volume subsides.

Each month deductions against each specialty pool must also be applied, before the pool is paid out to physicians. Such deductions may include in-area referrals to non-network physicians, fee-for-service carve-outs, and other negotiated items. The deductions against the specialty pool can substantially affect the contact yield if such deductions are large. Physicians should be concerned as to how such chargebacks are applied and by whom. For example, if a primary care physician consistently refers to a non-contact capitated specialist, those fee-for-service payments to that physician will be charged back to the specialty pool. The IPA should identify primary care physicians who routinely engage in such referral behavior, and work to correct the problem.

Another potential complication emerged when a payer introduced a low option product with higher copays and certain benefit restrictions. The IPA leadership was asked whether contact capitation should differentiate between products. The argument for differentiation was that the contacts with higher copays meant that a physician was getting overpaid for those low option patients if the contacts were not adjusted. The counter-response before the IPA leadership was that the low option patients could access the same network, and all physicians would be seeing these patients. Therefore, all physicians would be equally overpaid for those patients, thereby canceling out any benefit to a particular physician. The IPA ultimately decided to count the low option contacts in the same manner as the high option contacts. Had they decided otherwise, the low option contacts would have been weighted less than the high option contacts to adjust for the higher copays under the low option product. Either way was fair. To count all contacts the same was just easier to implement and administer.

FUTURE ENHANCEMENTS

Contact capitation has helped align physician incentives, but additional capabilities in this area would allow for greater sensitivity to market- and case-specific anomalies. Retrospective outpatient severity adjustment and prospective severity adjustment on a statistically reliable basis are enhancements that would increase the sophistication of the payment method. Currently, severity adjustment is handled through a collaborative Delphi technique of local physician experts. Validating that judgment statistically and being able to prospectively predict expected resource consumption would allow more refined severity adjustments to contact capitation.

Contact capitation can serve as a foundation for implementing or expanding disease management programs. Contact capitation is a payment method particularly suited to chronic care management and physicians will be more receptive to initiatives that help them and their patients manage their conditions. With contact capitation, physicians are more interested in patient compliance with therapeutic regimens such as physical therapy, exercise, weight management, prescription drug use, and psychosocial coping with their disease process.

Contact capitation encourages physicians to find and adopt best practices within their specialty. To the extent that physicians can be more effective in their clinical practice, with contact capitation they directly benefit from the clinical improvements they make.

SUGGESTED READINGS

Frank, C. 1999. Contact Capitation for Specialists. *Cost & Quality Quarterly Journal* 5, No. 2: 34–36.

Frank, C. and Roeder, R. 1999. Specialty Contact Capitation. *Journal of Health Care Finance* 25, No. 3: 17–21.

1998. Contact capitation: The coming craze for specialists. *Capitation Management Report* 5, No. 5: 1–6.

1998. Orthopedics presents new wrinkle in contact capitation. *Capitation Management Report* 5, No. 8: 120–123.

1999. *Medical Network Strategy Report*, May, 108.

1999. Profile network performance to manage contact capitation. *Capitation Management Report* 6, No. 5: 72–77.

CHAPTER 4

Keeping Close to Your Patients through Capitated Medicare

Fred C. Campbell, Jr., MD, FACP

Dr. Fred Campbell is an Internist in the San Antonio area. He has practiced there for 15 years. He is a former medical director for a large local HMO and has served on two National Formulary committees and Regional Advisory committees. He is currently in a primary care medical group of 15 serving over 10,000 managed care patients.

In this environment, he has had a great deal of success in managing a Medicare population in a capitated environment. He has personally cared for up to 700 managed Medicare patients at a time and maintained hospital day rates of one-third traditional Medicare rates.

To gain from his experience, we've asked Dr. Campbell to share his insights and several patient cases that exemplify approaches to managing in a Medicare capitated environment.

Describe How You Feel Working in a Capitated Managed Care Environment Compared to Fee-For-Service

I have made a career working in managed care for several important reasons:

- My experience with observing traditional medical care, something I call "unmanaged care" led me to believe that this mode of practice was a downward spiral into higher and higher health care costs without a higher level of quality. There have been ample examples of ordering inappropriate tests without clear rationale and performing unnecessary procedures such as hysterectomies, carotid endarterectomies, coronary artery bypass grafts to name a few that frequently cannot be proven to improve a patient's quality of life and often placed patients at some risk. "Defensive medicine" or the practice of ordering unnecessary tests to defend oneself in court was to me irrational and frequently not based on predetermined best practice algorithms. Traditional fee-for-service is conducive to such fraudulent practices as self-referral schemes, kickback schemes, and other examples of fraud especially in the Medicare area in dealing with a large federal bureaucracy.

- My dream was to organize small medical groups that worked cohesively together in a fully integrated practice, taking responsibility for both the medical care and financial risk for a population of patients. Preventive care using established algorithms for diagnosis and treatment and establishing optimum days of institutional care for elective procedures and other medical diagnoses could actually improve overall medical quality, preserve patient satisfaction, and ensure a steady reasonable level of compensation for me and my colleagues. Ultimately, being dictated to by outside parties who held purse strings for the care of my patients was undesirable as opposed to controlling my patients' destiny and my financial future as well.

How Does Actual Clinicians' Experience Working in This Capitated Environment Compare with Their Expectations? Describe the Emotions of Clinicians with Whom You Have Worked in This Environment

Quality is the *sine qua non* in selecting colleagues with whom to practice in a capitated, fully integrated environment. Without such essentials as good prior training, practical experience, board certification, and a commitment to continuing medical education, all other endeavors are difficult if not impossible. Some of my colleagues have had prior managed care experience; others are fresh out of training with some expectations but no bad habits from practicing in a fee-for-service environment. The key area in which emotional upheaval can occur is peer review. This typically occurs during weekly meetings to consider the status of our institutionalized patients and also on a retrospective basis as we attempt to audit our medical practice in a systematic fashion though utilization review and quality assurance committees. Some physicians shy away from this degree of scrutiny, but in general a well-selected group of individuals working closely together realizes that this is the only way effective patient care can be accomplished in a fully capitated and integrated setting. Likewise, they understand that shared responsibility for efficient practice will lead to increasing financial rewards over time. A close working relationship is conducive to improvement in quality of life in that we work closely together to satisfy each other's expectations regarding leave requests and personal emergencies.

Could You Give an Example of a Medically Complicated Clinical Case and How You Would Approach Managing It under Capitation?

Scene: Intensive care unit in your hospital

A 75-year-old widowed female, diabetic, smoker with a history of ischemic heart disease, has had operative repair of her left femur fracture 30 days ago. She had a myocardial infarction postoperatively, 2 days ago she developed fever associated with a sacral decubitus ulcer. Blood culture from 2 days ago was positive for Staph aureus, Methacillin-resistant. She would require intubation today for evidence of respiratory failure and sepsis syndrome. Past history of note is that she has had diabetes for 20 years with numerous complications and a similar smoking history. She apparently fell at night 1 month ago getting up for the bathroom and was found by a friend the next morning. She has one son, an attorney, who lives out of state and has not been in close contact. She depends on a long-term friend and companion who lives nearby. This case is an all too familiar one for primary care physicians who treat Medicare-age patients. The following is a systematic sequence of interventions of a preventive nature exemplifying a fully integrated practice mode with Medicare patients. (See Exhibit 4–1 which details the integration review process.)

Day T—1 day

This extremely high-risk case requires the highest-level subspecialty consultation at the first sign of fever or infection in order to avert catastrophic complications; specifically an infectious disease consultant should direct diagnosis and treatment. Ancillary consultation such as a wound care specialist for the decubitus ulcers and other physical therapy services would be appropriate.

Exhibit 4–1 The Integration Review Process

The key to cost-effective integrated medical care in a globally capitated payment system rests in the weekly patient care committee involved in concurrent utilization review. This body consists of all primary care physicians in a small medical group or a subgroup of primary care physicians in a much larger group. This may also include subspecialists within that group, if any. Administrative support includes one or more resource utilization nurses (also referred to as case manager nurses) and their clerical support including individuals who process and coordinate referrals. The process typically begins with a review of current acute hospital patients and patients in skilled nursing facilities with a discussion of their clinical condition and optimal care plan, including estimated lengths of stay and support needed to move from one setting to another. Second, a review of elective procedures is done, including more controversial procedures such as podiatry services, borderline cosmetic procedures such as rhinoplasty or other ENT, and oral surgery procedures. Concurrent review of the quality and cost effectiveness of consultants and ancillary facilities can be done on an informal basis at that time.

Subcommittee work in an integrated system should include ongoing proactive work in both the utilization review and quality improvement areas. Primary care and specialty physicians can work in their areas of interest and expertise. Utilization review should focus on adequacy of providing preventive services such as mammography, other routine screening, completeness of the medical record for these specific services, review of length of stay for specific surgical procedures such as total hip replacement or coronary artery bypass surgery, and referral rates in high cost, high volume areas, e.g., cardiology, radiology, orthopedic surgery, etc.

A quality improvement subcommittee is required to concentrate first and foremost on a systematic approach to preventive services, including immunization, cancer screening, coronary risk reduction screening, and other appropriate areas utilizing the latest expert recommendations from national and world organizations. Compliance with these recommendations can be audited by either a utilization or quality improvement process. Secondarily, but of comparable importance, is the development of clinical guidelines for common outpatient problems including such areas as optimum treatment of urinary tract infections, sinusitis, diabetes, and hypertension. Consultation with frequently used specialists in these areas is encouraged and can lead to

continues

Exhibit 4–1 continued

> improved relationships with consultants. This exercise also allows for a focused review of competence among consulting groups. Ultimately, shared information from utilization review and quality improvement subcommittees may allow a primary care physician group to subcapitate with specific subspecialty groups on the basis of quality and cost-effective practice.

Day T—1 week

This high-risk scenario of a recent myocardial in-farction in a postoperative patient with obligatory bed confinement should prompt prophylactic intervention that may extend beyond the usual hospital support. Specifically, the order of a specialty bed to increase patient mobility and decrease the incidence of decubitus ulcer is clearly indicated. Consultation with a clinical medical specialist or a trained physical therapist in the hospital to maximize physical activity is highly desirable.

Day T—3 weeks

Postoperative myocardial infarction could be successfully managed by a primary care physician; however, recent studies suggest strongly that early cardiology consultation is associated with improved prognosis in the setting of an acute myocardial infarction. Appropriate arrangements for hospital care including a routine use of a "hospitalist" or intensivist familiar with both cardiac and pulmonary intensive care would be reasonable alternatives.

Day T—6 weeks

Elderly patients are at high risk for falls and hip fractures and are candidates for an intensive program in short-term preventive techniques such as:

- a systematic physical therapy program of proactive gait assessment and training
- attention to visual acuity and prompt referral for refraction
- a contractual arrangement with visiting nurses or a systematic program by a case manager nurse to conduct home safety evaluations
- implementation of a program to review "high-risk" medications associated with increased fall risk and alerting of practitioners who care for these patients

Day T—1 year

Long-term preventive strategies pertinent to this case include the following:

- a systemically devised program of aggressive medical therapy of Type 2 diabetes with particular attention to prevention of complications including routine eye screening and early referral of peripheral neuropathy for gate training and maintenance
- an integrated approach to reduction of risk factors for atherosclerosis including aggressive medical treatment of hypertension, hyperlipidemia, and a systematic smoking cessation program including pharmaceutical support
- aggressive preventive therapy of osteoporosis including traditional estrogen replacement therapy and/or newer pharmacological approaches such as Alendronate. Proactive wellness programs should also be provided by the medical group or in conjunction with the affiliated managed care plan
- routine education of higher risk individuals and assisted living or various living assistive devices such as various forms of transferring aids
- early discussion of advance directives including health care proxy and provision of standard forms in conjunction with medical societies and hospice programs

Would You Describe What the Peer Interactions Are Like in This Integration Process?

With the understanding that being involved in a group over a long period of time is the most effective way of realizing the rewards of a fully integrated practice, my colleagues and I work in a very collegial fashion for the most part. We tend to use each other's expertise and experience in various areas of medical care to augment other colleagues' capabilities in taking care of patients. For instance, we may teach skills such as casting or joint injection to improve our technical capability. Additionally, we frequently share information from recent continuing education, experiences, or journal reading as to the latest developments in diagnoses and therapy during the course of our weekly integration review committee process.

Animated debates do occur on a frequent basis, especially regarding such areas as the concept of medical necessity when it comes to certain types of procedures. For example, breast reduction surgery can be supported on medical grounds but these are highly subjective and subject to question. The use of consultants, who are more costly or out of our geographic area, because of their level of expertise has also led to a great amount of debate over appropriateness. Ultimately, we may actually need to take a vote to resolve issues discussed, especially when they deal with personal issues outside the strict area of medical care. A recent example of this was a young college student who developed Hodgkin's disease and was also the son of two local physicians. They requested that he continue his chemotherapy at his college environment in Georgia. A compromise had to be ironed out between the use of oncology consultants of the patient's choice and a much more economical system within the contractual boundaries of their insurance plan. Frequently we will convince each other that a more expensive procedure or consultant not only is better for patient care but also is also more economical in the long term. As you can imagine, there is a tension between short-term expenditures on certain procedures and equipment and long-term outcomes and efficiency.

Among the most heated discussions is what are the minimum standards for screening, for example, the recommendations regarding screening mammography. The strong emotional and political overlay related to this topic has led to resolutions by Congress in support of screening intervals that may or may not have had medical support. We must be meticulous in our review of the medical literature to satisfy our colleagues, our patients, and optimize the financial investment in the area of prevention. Our narrow screening recommendations regarding mammography are believed to be sound from an academic standpoint but may not be satisfying to all our gynecological or surgical colleagues. We undoubtedly will be required to defend them at some point in a medical-legal forum and feel confident of being able to do so.

Could You Give an Example of Your Best and Worst Consultant Interactions?

Unquestionably the "golden list" for us is our reliable and competent consultants. Optimally, there should be several groups to choose from within a particular specialty so that competition will encourage cooperation. Quality is our most important selection criteria for specialists, including willingness to participate in continuing medical education and to teach our own group from time to time in a formal setting as well as in informal ways. Locally, consultant groups have evolved from a position of antagonism toward managed care practices and a superior position in demanding fees to one of increased competition for patients and a high degree of willingness to negotiate both discounted rates in a fee-for-service mode and also subcapitation agreements. This has been to a great extent a financial necessity but has also occurred because of the stability of physician groups practicing in a primary care capitated mode over a period of greater than 10 years. Subcapitation arrangements are worth looking at but are not necessarily more financially or practically desirable than a well-negotiated discounted fee-for-service arrangement. Subcapitation requires a high degree of cooperation between the primary care and consulting groups, especially in the care of more complex medical problems. Confrontation over quality issues as well as utilization of resources is best resolved retrospectively through the committee process and intergroup meetings rather than at the time being delivered; however, patient safety may dictate a change of consultant on a more urgent basis.

One of the most distressing circumstances occurred following several years of subcapitation with one cardiology subspecialty group that was involved in the care of large numbers of our group's capitated patients. If there are serious concerns over quality, utilization of resources, or both, transfer of care to another consulting group must occur in a systemic and deliberate fashion to ensure both continuity and also satisfaction from the patients' standpoint. On one occasion, the full transition from one cardiology consulting group to another required approximately two years of deliberate case-by-case decision making. Alternatively, using several groups to perform cardiology consultation in a discounted fee-for-service arrangement would be less likely to lead to such a painful and difficult transition.

Conflicts over resource utilization such as the length of stay for a patient after elective surgery can usually be discussed and resolved in an amicable fashion through intergroup discussions. However, circumstances do develop where highly technical procedures performed by only one or two individuals within the community may be required. In that circumstance, a primary group is at the mercy of that consultant to determine both the type and the course of therapy. The only way to influence utilization of resources would be to compare national or international standards of care with the performance of that particular consultant to establish deviations from norms. This can require a high degree of diplomacy and tact and is frequently unsuccessful as the consultant has a local "monopoly" on this procedure or technique.

What's Another Clinical Case Regarding a Medicare Senior That Focuses Largely on Surgical Care and Reflects Your Approach to Care Management?

Scene: Surgical ward at your local hospital

An 80-year-old otherwise healthy man has undergone a left total knee replacement one week ago. The orthopedic consultant has told the patient that he will need a "rehabilitation hospital" for extended physical therapy. The patient's discharge has already been delayed by three days by an episode of light leg pain that led to a positive duplex scan of that leg from deep venous thrombosis on postoperative Day 4. The patient's wife wants "the best facility in town" for rehabilitation; her mother died in a nursing home years ago from what she perceives as woefully inadequate care. The following is an outline of preventive strategies to reduce the likelihood of the above scenario.

Day T—7 days

Consultant choice is key to optimal surgical and postoperative medical management of the case in question; it is also essential to controlling facility costs. Notwithstanding surgical quality, the orthopedist is expected to know about and use standard prophylactic therapy of deep venous thrombosis of such postoperative patients, decreasing the risk of this life-threatening complication and typically shortening the stay in an acute care facility.

Day T—30 days

As soon as this elective surgery is deemed necessary, a resource utilization nurse (also referred to as a case manager nurse) should undertake a proactive coordination of the patient's overall care strategy, including:

- Heading up a meeting with the patient and family to outline specifically which facilities will be used and the estimated length of stay at each, including the duration of home care, if any

- Setting up visits to facilities in advance for the patient and family, including an outpatient physical therapy facility if it is to be used
- Ensuring that the recommended preoperative laboratory tests are completed in a timely and cost-effective manner
- Verifying with the proposed consultant or consultants that the agreed-upon facilities, length of stay, and testing are acceptable

Day T—180 days

An ongoing relationship between the primary care group and the preferred orthopedic group should be fostered in order to manage degenerative joint disease effectively for prevention of premature total knee replacements, including agreement on timing of interarticular steroid injections and the use of arthroscopy.

Day T—2 years

A routine assessment of prospective skilled nursing facilities directed by the resource utilization nurse in conjunction with both the primary care group and the preferred orthopedic group should be conducted to ensure:

- Optimum physical therapy capability and access such as performance of services on weekends and multiple times during the day
- Access to admissions on a 24-hours-a-day 7-days-a-week basis from hospitals and emergency rooms
- The highest level of overall capability and quality control including the administration of intravenous medications and local wound care

A similar assessment of acute hospital support should be conducted on an ongoing basis by the medical groups with education from the physical therapy programs in these facilities as to the optimum length of stay and level of physical therapy for elective cases.

Last, an easily accessible program of safe moderate levels of physical activity should be available to the appropriate patient population as part of a systematic preventive program.

Describe a Resource Utilization Nurse Who Particularly Epitomizes the Position. Describe Him or Her Personally.

Cheryl S., RN is in her early 40s. She began college in 1977 but suspended her education to have a family and now has adult children. She received her

RN in San Antonio in 1990; thereafter, she had a critical care residency in 1991 in a local hospital. She spent an additional year in intensive care units in a tertiary hospital. For the following three years she was an RN field nurse and clinical supervisor for a home health nursing company and has been a resource utilization nurse (case manager; Exhibit 4–2) with our medical group since 1995.

Cheryl is highly personable and vivacious and has an unlimited amount of enthusiasm for her work and for the people around her, especially her patients. She has the respect and affection of her physician colleagues in our medical group as well as in consultant groups. She is tactful and diplomatic in working with consultants and patients alike in suggesting alternatives to prolonged hospital stays, especially following elective surgery. She has an instinctive knack for anticipating the need for clinical services following hospital discharge and can triage patients effectively to various levels of skilled care, both in nursing facilities and through home care agencies.

She acts as the extension of our primary care physicians to home care, skilled nursing care, hospital care outside of geographic area, and to various ancillary agencies such as suppliers of durable medical equipment. She continually monitors the quality of acute hospitals, skilled nursing facilities, home care agencies, suppliers of durable medical equipment, and hospice agencies as she makes her daily rounds; only someone with her extensive and varied clinical experience would be able to accomplish this task effectively. She communicates the need for changes in support services to our physician group through participation in our regular patient care committee meetings.

Resource utilization nurses such as Cheryl are indispensable to integrated clinical practice and make practitioners infinitely more efficient. Cheryl will return to college in the fall to receive her bachelor of science in nursing and will take a certification exam as a nurse case manager this summer.

How Do Physicians Respond to Physician Extenders?

Among the most effective enhancements in an integrated practice is the appropriate use of physician extenders. A recent example is the use of a nurse practitioner to provide all diabetic education and devise a system for monitoring the efficiency of control of our diabetic population. This

Exhibit 4–2 Resource Utilization Nurse

The position of resource utilization nurse (also known as case manager nurse) is pivotal to the successful integration of a globally capitated primary care practice. These nurses serve as the proxy for primary care physicians during busy patient care sessions and ensure that physicians' arrangements for cost-effective care are executed properly. Qualification for these individuals include a minimum registered nurse level of education and training, and optimally a bachelor's degree. Experience includes an extensive background in clinical medicine including acute hospital patient responsibility and optimally supervisory responsibility as well. These nurses should demonstrate a level of comfort with confronting physicians regarding utilization issues and must display a high level of tact and diplomacy. They must have a clear understanding of the goals of an integrated practice and demonstrate an instinct for recognizing potential overutilization of institutional days by avoidable delays in accomplishing procedures, for instance, and be ready with contingency plans to circumvent these delays. Ultimately, they must consider themselves partners with the physician group working toward a common goal of the optimum cost-effective practice.

Responsibilities of resource utilization nurses include the following:

1. Continuous monitoring of hospital and skilled nursing facility patients with frequent interaction with primary care physicians and consultants to minimize unnecessary bed days in these facilities.

2. Coordination of smooth transition between more acute and less acute patient care situations such as between a hospital and skilled nursing facility or skilled nursing facility and home care. This responsibility includes a proactive plan of education of patients and consultants as to the likely length of stay for elective procedures and transition to less acute levels of care.

3. Continuous evaluation of the quality and utilization practices of acute care hospitals, rehabilitation hospitals, skilled nursing facilities, home nursing agencies, hospice programs, and outpatient surgical facilities, providing regular feedback to utilization and quality improvement committees within an integrated primary care practice.

continues

Exhibit 4–2 continued

4. Assessment of cost effectiveness of various medical suppliers including durable medical equipment.

5. Ongoing assessment of the practice consultants as to quality of care, accessibility, responsiveness to comments on optimum utilization of facilities and services, and overall cooperation. Resource utilization nurses are typically supported by clerical managed care specialists who coordinate the execution of referrals and follow-up care.

individual has the experience, expertise, and personal interest to specialize in this vital area of our practice and interact well with both patients and primary physicians within our group. Conversely, a physician extender who fails to practice by established protocols devised by and monitored by the group would quickly get into trouble and lose support on the part of the physicians. One classic example is the physician extender's overuse of antibiotics to treat typical viral illnesses at a time where most physicians are attempting to minimize unnecessary antibiotic use. Patient expectation may pressure a mid-level practitioner into a poor practice decision for the purpose of maintaining his or her popularity as a practitioner; this could lead to disastrous consequences for both the practitioner and patient. In my experience, the best situation with mid-level practitioners is where that individual performs one particular type of service on an ongoing basis, making physicians within the group much more efficient.

What Is Going On with Prescription Drugs?

The area of financial responsibility for prescription drugs by a medical group is a highly complex one and evolves over an extended period of time. Factors completely outside the area of medical care such as competition among health plans in the area of prescription benefits can significantly affect the financial desirability of risk assumption in this area. Having said that, I believe that there is great potential for improving the quality of practice and the cost effectiveness of prescribing prescription drugs by several simple techniques:

- Educating both primary care physicians and consultants as to the most cost-effective representatives in each therapeutic class of pharmaceuticals

- Continuing education as to newer therapeutic alternatives that are improvements in management of certain disorders, for example the treatment of peptic ulcer disease with antibiotic regimens designed to eradicate H. Pylori bacteria
- Providing regular critical feedback to formulary committees of major health plans in appraisal of more expensive agents in a therapeutic category
- Working with health plans to audit the most expensive drugs used by a physician group over time to determine if those drugs are being used appropriately and for the appropriate length of time
- Working toward a system of providing effective over-the-counter equivalents to more expensive prescription drugs in treatment of self-limited conditions

Is There an Example of "Unmanaged Care" To Contrast with What You've Shared Already?

Jane Doe is a 65-year-old female who presents to your office for preoperative evaluation prior to nasal septal surgery recommended by ENT.

Ms. Doe was seen originally four months earlier by a "diet specialist" in the community and prescribed a thyroid medication to assist her in weight loss. After six weeks of this regimen, she developed severe palpitations and lightheadedness and was evaluated at a local emergency room. The evaluation revealed atrial fibrillation, and the patient was referred to a cardiologist on call. Digitalis and Warfarin were prescribed to prevent a stroke. The patient refused to reveal her diet pills due to embarrassment, but discontinued them after discharge from the hospital. She felt better and did not return to her cardiologist but continued to take both Digoxin and Warfarin. Six weeks later she developed a profuse right-sided nosebleed and again was seen in the emergency room. She was found to have a prolonged prothrombin time due to Warfarin excess, which was reversed with plasma. She was evaluated by an ENT specialist who packed her bleeding nostril and recommended follow-up in the office. Upon return to the ENT's office, she underwent nasal endoscopy to rule out malignancy. This procedure was negative, but the specialist recommended a nasal septal repair to "help her breathe better." She was referred to you for preoperative medical evaluation prior to elective septoplasty. Your examination reveals a well-appearing elderly female without evidence of atrial fibrillation and with a normal appearing nasal septum. She sheepishly reveals the thyroid hormone tablets that she had been given originally for weight loss.

DISCUSSION

Although many patients will go outside the medical community to obtain questionable medications, a long-term consistent relationship with a primary care physician frequently will dissuade individuals from alternative medical care. An integrated medical practice with easy access to consulting dieticians can provide patients with a healthy alternative for success in long-term weight reduction. The approach to the patient's secondary atrial fibrillation was appropriate including the use of anticoagulation to prevent stroke; however patients are too frequently reluctant to follow up with a new consultant for necessary monitoring of their anticoagulation status. This leads to complications such as the one in the above case history and even more life-threatening situations. Evaluation of nosebleed does not ordinarily involve full endoscopy on an otherwise healthy individual. The use of ENT consultants often leads to a recommendation to provide patients with elective cosmetic procedures that may have no impact on their health status. An experienced primary care physician can manage the course of nosebleed with frequent office visits, obviating the need for expensive and unnecessary further investigation. Coordination and proper direction of medical care is the hallmark of a well-designed and integrated medical practice in a capitated payment system.

As You Think about the Experiences and Cases That You've Shared, What Are the Core Themes of Your Success in Managing a Capitated Medicare Population?

- Gaining a critical mass of patients and having their care provided by a selective group of practitioners is very important. For example, 300–700 patients/month is workable depending on other responsibilities.
- Operating in a positive, group practice environment with respected colleagues is also critical. In the right group environment, you learn together, support each other logistically, and have an open dialogue

about thorny, often sensitive patient care and coverage issues. I can't imagine working nearly as effectively without that.

- The linkage to the right specialty consultants is invaluable for the sake of cost-effective care, good communication, problem solving, trust, and continuing education. Many complex cases can develop into both cost and quality nightmares without the cooperation of good specialty consultants.

- Good care management requires a team approach that encompasses the primary care physician, consultants, physician extenders, nurses, support staff, and the patient. Roles need to be defined well so that all persons on the team know how they contribute to the care of the patient or member. At the same time, there needs to be enough flexibility to respond to newly developing circumstances. Traditionally, much emphasis is placed on the physician, but in our system, for example, the resource utilization nurse plays a very pivotal role in good care management.

- Developing "small" simple systems to support patient care management is also very important. Often, so much emphasis is placed on automation and overall integration. We have developed files, templates, flow charts, reminder and follow-up systems, and case notes, among many tools, to enable successful care management. Over time, we have standardized and automated, but that has been secondary to getting tools in play on behalf of our patients and ourselves.

- Finally, it all comes down to good patient care planning. So much of medical care, today, is still handled on an ad hoc, episodic basis. Due to the incentives of capitation, we focus a lot of attention on prevention, education, and early intervention with our patients. That requires more on our part on the front end, but it pays off, in my opinion, in better care, health improvement, lower costs, and predictability. I see health care delivery in the capitated environment as a wonderful exercise, but one that never forgets the personal considerations of our patients.

SUGGESTED READINGS

Eddy, D.M. 1994. Rationing Resources while Improving Quality. *The Journal of the American Medical Association* 272: 817–824.

Fawles, J.B. et al. 1996. Taking Health Status into Account when Setting Capitation Rates. *The Journal of the American Medical Association* 276: 1316–1321.

Fisher, E.S. et al. 1999. Avoiding the Unintended Consequences of Growth in Medical Care. *The Journal of the American Medical Association* 281: 446–454.

Kassirer, J. 1995. Managed Care and the Morality of the Marketplace. *The New England Journal of Medicine* 333: 50–52.

Mirvis, D.M. et al. 1997. Managing Care, Managing Uncertainity. *Archives of Internal Medicine* 157: 385–388.

Simson, S.R. et al. 1999. View of Managed Care. *The New England Journal of Medicine* 340: 928–936.

Woolhandler, S. et al. 1995. Extreme Risk—The New Corporate Proposition for Physicians. *The New England Journal of Medicine* 333: 1706–1708.

Chapter 5

Medicaid Capitation— Tag, You're It!

Joel Hornberger, MHS

The room was silent as the executive staff of Healthtron arrived for a special "called" meeting. Two days earlier, the anemic balance sheet of this multispecialty physician group practice had been distributed with a terse handwritten note by the CEO: "Let's discuss ASAP." What had once been a thriving, 42-physician practice only nine months earlier was now rapidly crashing and burning. Cash had plummeted. Accounts receivables had skyrocketed. Payables were overdue. Payroll was on Friday. Blood was on the boardroom floor, and everyone knew it.

At exactly 7 AM, Dr. Janice Kaplan, Healthron's CEO, entered the Board Room and took her seat at the head of the long oval table. She was a careful executive, always asking penetrating questions—not to hurt or embarrass, but to understand and repair her damaged company. Her lieutenants knew this was going to be a long day. Dr. Kaplan was going to get to the bottom of the problems. As they fidgeted nervously in their seats, they just hoped they were not identified as the problem.

"Good morning. I take it you have all seen our latest financial statements." Dr. Kaplan rarely minced words. Nods and throat-clearing indicated that they had. "How did we get here?" she asked.

Everyone knew that Dr. Kaplan would never ask such an open-ended question unless she had a very good idea of the answer, but she seemed to genuinely want their input.

"Two words—Managed Medicaid," said Josh Horn, CFO. He was always outspoken, but had the financial brilliance to back it up.

"Go on," said Dr. Kaplan.

"Well, ever since the State turned over the Medicaid program to the private Managed Care Organizations, we've been getting killed. Some of the MCOs pay us ridiculously low capitation rates and others pay us ridiculously low fee-for-service rates. And those that pay us capitation keep saying 'Oh, that's included in the cap rate' whenever we question a fee-for-service denial. To top it off, we're not getting any eligibility reports with our cap checks—just the checks. We have no idea who's in, who's out, or when they became eligible. And on the fee-for-service side, the MCOs either don't know how to pay claims within 30 days or they're so swamped with hundreds of thousands of members that they're just buried in claims." Josh was clearly angry.

"Have we talked to the MCOs? What about their Provider Relations Reps? Can they help us?" asked Dr. Kaplan.

Dr. Montrose, the group's Medical Director, spoke up, "*Everyone* is screaming at them. They hired so many so fast that they haven't been trained. They're mostly recent college grads with degrees in horticulture! The only thing they know about managed Medicaid is to say 'I'm sorry, that's not covered.' They're not very helpful."

"That's for sure!" exclaimed Al Holt, General Counsel for the group. "I've tried everything to get them to address these problems—even threatening to sue them. They are just unresponsive. They say we have to arbitrate."

"Okay, okay," Dr. Kaplan said. "Now before we all have strokes, let's look at these problems one by one."

"We'll be here 'til Christmas if we're going to do that!" joked Josh. Those in the room chuckled and nodded in agreement.

"Then I hope you have your shopping done, Josh, because we're not leaving here until we've gone over this mess." Dr. Kaplan was not amused. "Okay," she said, "let's back up. Al, give us the background on how we got here—managed Medicaid in the State."

Al cleared his throat and spoke, "As you all know, the State decided to 'privatize' the State's Medicaid program last year. The State was going broke with 15–20 percent budget increases each year for the last four or five years. Medicaid was killing them. Inpatient costs were climbing. Pharmacy was going through the roof. Alcohol and drug costs were adding up as patients went in and out of rehab. The governor started screaming. So the legislature started screaming."

Al paused for effect. "They had three choices: (1) raise taxes, (2) cut benefits and/or beneficiaries, or (3) manage the costs of the program through managed care companies. Privatize it. Raising taxes would tick off everyone in the State, and they'd vote everyone out of office. Cutting benefits or beneficiaries would tick off the 1.5 million Medicaid beneficiaries and all the bleeding hearts in the State, who, by the way, also vote. The average taxpayer didn't care if they balanced the budget by reducing payments to 'rich' doctors and hospitals. So the only smart thing for them to do politically was to manage the costs. So that's how we got here."

"Yeah, but is anyone really 'managing' the program costs? Didn't they really just 'cap' the costs for the State? No one's really managing the program," asked Josh angrily.

"That's true, Josh. It's a very important point," continued Al. "The State said 'this dollar amount is all we're going to pay' for the program. They 'capped' it at their budget level, and that's all they're going to pay. It's up to the managed care organizations to provide the benefits within that budget. They took the costs of the Medicaid program for the last couple of years, divided by the number of enrollees, and came up with what they call a 'capitation' rate. It's an idiot's guide to capitation."

"I remember something about an actuary coming up with the rates," Dr. Kaplan stated.

"People forget that actuarial science is really 'actuarial art' when it comes to Medicaid," said Josh.

"More like actuarial smoke and mirrors," said Al.

Josh continued, "Yes, for commercial HMO business they know their stuff. They have decent utilization data, pricing information, enrollee estimates—decent data. They're good at commercial rating. But Medicaid is another story. They don't have good claims history, and the State used to do all its own claims processing. Their focus was on paying claims, not on building a reliable database. Nobody thought that far ahead. So the actuaries have really struggled with 'pricing' the Medicaid benefit package. I'd say the rates are an educated guess with enough smoke and mirrors to make them fly politically."

"They've never published any actuarial analysis that we providers have seen," stated Al.

"Go on, Al," said Dr. Kaplan.

"Well, as I said, the State had to privatize the program. There was too much at stake politically to not do it. So the State put out a 'Request for Proposal' and all the big national managed care organizations and all the little local guys jumped on it. Now remember, the State bureaucrats have zero experience doing this." Al was quickening his pace as he spoke on one of his favorite subjects.

"But didn't they have help? HCFA and consultants?" asked Dr. Kaplan.

"Yes, they had to get a waiver from HCFA.[1] But how hard is that to do? HCFA even gave a waiver to Tennessee, for crying out loud! You have to remember that managed Medicaid is first and foremost a political decision with economic consequences. It is not the other way around. Politics drives the machinery of 'privatized' Medicaid."

Al was hitting his stride. "So, because the State bureaucrats know so little about true managed care, they have become increasingly co-opted by the MCOs. Only the MCOs have 'experience' managing care. The MCOs exert more and more power, and get their way in contract negotiations with the State."

Dr. Kaplan took a deep breath and summarized, "Okay, so we got here because the State had to privatize Medicaid. And the capitation rates are best guesses because of poor quality data. And the MCOs are running the show. Right?" Everyone nodded in agreement.

"So tell me this," Dr. Kaplan continued, "if we knew all this a year ago, why did we sign an agreement with these people? Why did we agree to 'ridiculously low capitation rates,' Josh?"

"Well, it wasn't really a negotiation. They said these are the rates, take them or leave them. It's all we have budgeted."

"Why didn't we leave them?" asked Dr. Kaplan.

Josh was clearly irked by the question and looked around the room. "I think we all know why. We've had a mission to the Medicaid population for over 20 years. They represent over 50 percent of our historic income. We thought the MCOs would be fair. So there wasn't much doubt that we would walk."

Dr. Kaplan recalled the "negotiations" very clearly and knew Josh was correct. She had preached "Mission, Mission, Mission," and Josh had argued "Margin, Margin, Margin." She knew that was why Josh was irritated.

"Al," Dr. Kaplan said, "you said something a minute ago that interested me. You said we can't sue them?"

"That's right, our contract has an arbitration clause, which essentially makes us go that route rather than a lawsuit."

"Isn't that a better system?" asked Dr. Kaplan. "It's quicker, cheaper, and fair."

Al laughed. "That's the way it's supposed to be, but there are problems."

"Tell us about arbitration, then, Al," said Dr. Kaplan.

"Okay, first some background. Everyone knows that each year there are millions of business deals taking place. It's no surprise that some blow up, and the parties to the deal then have a dispute. Rather than going to court, many contracts have 'arbitration clauses' to provide a quicker, less costly, fair resolution to the dispute. One of the best organizations to use to arbitrate disputes is the American Arbitration Association (AAA). The AAA is a public service, not-for-profit organization. As its name suggests, it offers dispute services to nearly anyone needing their services—business executives, unions, attorneys, even families.

"Now here's the kicker though. The AAA's Standard Contract Arbitration Clause reads like this:"

> *Any controversy or claim arising out of or relating to this contract, or the breach thereof, shall be settled by arbitration administered by the American Arbitration Association under its Commercial Arbitration Rules, and judgment on the award rendered by the arbitrator(s) may be entered in any court having jurisdiction thereof.*[2]

"Our problem is that our contract has a different clause. The phrase 'administered by the American Arbitration Association under its Commercial Arbitration Rules' is missing, so ours reads:"

> *Any controversy or claim arising out of or relating to this contract, or the breach thereof, shall be settled by arbitration and judgment on the award rendered by the arbitrator(s) may be entered in any court having jurisdiction thereof.*

"So now the MCO is saying that we have to come up with an arbitration administrator and apply its rules, something they have simply stonewalled our doing. They won't agree to simply turn any disputes over to the AAA and allow the AAA to use their standard Commercial Arbitration Rules. It's a Catch-22. They say we can't take them to court; that we have to arbitrate, but we'll never be able to reach agreement on the arbitration administration or rules of arbitrating our dispute. A few words *not* in the contract, and we are now in a major mess over these claims, the cap rates, and everything else."

"How did we miss them?" asked Dr. Kaplan, somewhat irritably.

"We didn't," replied Al. "I pointed these out in my review of the contract, but the MCO said 'Take it or leave it.' We took it."

"That's outrageous! It's no wonder Medicaid can't find providers." Dr. Kaplan was visibly upset.

"What do these rules look like?" snapped Dr. Kaplan.

Al dug into his briefcase and produced the Commercial Arbitration Rules as Amended and Effective on July 1, 1996 published by the American Arbitration Association. "Here's what they look like," Al said and handed them to Dr. Kaplan.

Dr. Kaplan slowly scanned the heading of the Commercial Arbitration Rules and read a few of the rules[3]:

1. Agreement of Parties
2. Name of Tribunal
3. Administrator and Delegation of Duties
4. National Panel of Arbitrators
5. Regional Offices
6. Initiation under an Arbitration Provision in a Contract
7. Initiation under a Submission
8. Changes of Claim
9. Applicable Procedures
10. Administrative Conference, Preliminary Hearing, and Mediation Conference
11. Fixing of Locale
12. Qualifications of an Arbitrator
13. Appointment from Panel
14. Direct Appointment by a Party
15. Appointment of Neutral Arbitrator by Party-Appointed Arbitrators or Parties
16. Nationality of Arbitrator in International Arbitration
17. Number of Arbitrators
18. Notice to Arbitrator of Appointment
19. Disclosure and Challenge Procedure
20. Vacancies
21. Date, Time, and Place of Hearing
22. Representation
23. Stenographic Record
24. Interpreters
25. Attendance at Hearings
26. Postponements
27. Oaths

"Very comprehensive," Dr. Kaplan said. "I notice that we could submit any of our existing disputes over claims and capitation rates by employing the 'Submission' clause, if we could get the MCOs to agree to it."

We, the undersigned parties, hereby agree to submit to arbitration administered by the American Arbitration Association under its

Commercial Arbitration Rules the following controversy: (cite briefly). We further agree that the above controversy be submitted to (one) (three) arbitrator(s). We further agree that we will faithfully observe this agreement and the rules, that we will abide by and perform any award rendered by the arbitrator(s), and that a judgment of the court having jurisdiction may be entered on the award.

"It's certainly worth a shot," said Al. "It would give us the kind of clarification we need. But like you said, if the MCO would agree." Al scribbled down the clause on a yellow pad and made a note to enter into this negotiation.

"Okay, what's next. Let's see . . ." Dr. Kaplan said as she reviewed her notes. "Where are we on paid claims?"

Monica Evans, Director of Operations, spoke up. "We're getting a lot of denials. We thought the billed services were going to be paid under a fee-for-service reimbursement system, but they tell us the services are included in the capitation rate."

"How can that be?" asked Dr. Kaplan.

"Well, the contract has the capitation rate, but it doesn't have the procedure codes included in the rate. We should have asked them to spell out the procedure codes so we could tell what services were fee-for-service and what were capitated."

"Can we get those procedure codes now?" asked Josh.

"The MCO hasn't been forthcoming when I've asked for them. Things just keep getting lost whenever we ask for information," said Monica.

"Well, what's their problem?" exclaimed Dr. Kaplan. "Commercial MCOs don't have these problems!"

"We're all frustrated," said Josh, "but in fairness to them, they added 200,000 Medicaid eligible folks overnight—literally! A typical commercial HMO won't add that many people over several years. Imagine the strain on an already poorly functioning infrastructure. It's no wonder they can't pay claims, answer telephones, do UR, and so on."

"They had to meet the state contracting guidelines, didn't they? They should have the capability to handle their contract!" declared Dr. Kaplan.

"Yes, they should," said Al, "but remember what we said earlier—this managed Medicaid is political. It seems that few states are willing or able to address these problems. Look around at managed Medicaid. You see marketing fraud and abuse by some health plans, member education and enrollment processes in disarray, ineffective internal and external quality of care protections, the siphoning off of up to 30 percent of the state Medicaid payments for 'administrative' costs. . .the list goes on."

Josh agreed. "Has the State provided any meaningful oversight of the MCOs? Not much. They aren't checking the accuracy of data reported to it by the plans, making evaluation of the programs and plans impossible. We're seeing women giving birth who had no or inadequate prenatal care. We're seeing access to primary care docs declining and ER visits increasing threefold. We're seeing over 40 percent of preschool kids with Medicaid lacking all or part of their required medical exams. It's just that the State has no experience in monitoring managed care. They don't know what to look for most of the time and are incapable of effective monitoring even when they do. It's not just our State, just look at the journals—nearly every state is struggling."

"And because we have this mix of politics and dollars, you know the review process of the health plans is going to ensure their continuation. The State doesn't want any of the MCOs to drop out. Without the MCOs, there's no program. The State can't be too tough on the MCOs and make them perform or the MCOs might walk. If the Blues walk, the State's in big trouble, and the legislature is back to square one. So the attitude is, 'Relax, we'll fix things later. Rome wasn't built in a day. Trust us.' If you don't believe me, just look at the requirements laid out in the Balanced Budget Act, Information Standards, Marketing Prohibitions, Rules for enrollment brokers, HCFA's rules and proposed rules. . .shoot. . .Section 1902 of the Social Security Act,[4] and then compare that to what's going on! The State is either unwilling or unable to effectively monitor the program, pure and simple. You remember that even the Health Care Financing Administration and the General Accounting Office have found that 'the states' monitoring and oversight were often inadequate to ensure the provision of quality care to the Medicaid population.'"

"Several of you talked about eligibility issues," Dr. Kaplan said. "What's going on there?"

"That's a major problem. We're not getting eligibility files very consistently. Some months we get them with our cap check, but many others we don't. We just get the check," said Josh. "Even when we do get a printout or a disk of eligible people, I'd say 30 to 35 percent are wrong. Their eligibility has expired. We often treat Medicaid patients as well as the 'dual eligibles'—elderly or disabled covered under both Medicaid and Medicare—and then find out that the patients' eligibility has expired or they were never eligible in the first place. If the service was fee-for-service, we're getting denials in accounts receivable. If the service was included in the capitation, we never got paid the cap rate in the first place. Our docs are very busy, working their tails off, providing tons of free care. The lack of eligibility data is probably our most serious problem."

"Another problem," Josh continued, "is that now that the burden has been passed on to physicians, there's a screwy State provision that allows hospitals to place Medicaid patients into the plan retroactively—that is, *after* treating them. We're only finding out *after* the fact that a Medicaid patient who has just run up a huge hospital bill is in fact our patient, even though we've never laid eyes on the patient. Our hospital pool is dinged $10,000 to $20,000 per pop. It takes only a few of those to put us in the hole."

"How are we supposed to know who's eligible?" asked Dr. Kaplan.

"We don't. We just provide the care if a patient tells us they have Medicaid. Then we try to sort things out later."

"Wait a minute," Dr. Kaplan said. "Someone walks in the front door and says 'Hi, I'm in such and such HMO and on Medicaid,' and we just treat them? They don't even have to show us their Medicaid card?"

Josh smiled wearily. "Look, this population is tough. We're lucky they just show up. These are good people, but they're tough to deal with. For one thing, most of these people have never been in managed care before. They don't understand it. Some haven't had any kind of health care insurance for that matter. They don't understand the health care system—who does? The MCOs think their member education materials just need shorter words and more white space. They don't understand that it's very, very difficult to get members to understand and act on materials. When Medicaid members get letters, promotional brochures, member handbooks, forms, questionnaires, and other stuff from the MCOs, many don't read them. Don't even open them. The materials are culturally or linguistically wrong. So the Medicaid population is very different than a commercial HMO population that's employed and literate."

Josh continued. "To top that off, their addresses change constantly, so they don't even get the stuff mailed to them, including ID cards. Many don't have telephones so we can't call to remind them of their appointments. Transportation is a continuous problem for most so we have a 40 percent no-show rate, and if we double-book appointments and everyone *does* show up, the docs get upset. Most of the time these folks are dealing with multiple, serious medical or mental health conditions—this is a very resource-intensive population. They don't have access to or money for child care so they have to bring all the kids along with them, and either leave them unattended in the waiting room or bring them along in and want them seen by the doc too. The last thing many are thinking about is their ID card—about 50 percent of the time. So we see them and hope they're ours."

"But getting back to eligibility—the problems of eligibility would be a lot less if the State allowed a full year of eligibility for Medicaid recipients and required the person to stay with the same PCP for the whole time—like in Tennessee. They didn't do much right, but they did get that one right. But here, we have six months eligibility and the patient is allowed to change PCPs monthly if they want to. The Feds require "freedom of choice" for patients under Section 1902, and the State has interpreted that to mean they can change primary care physicians every 30 days. The State has refused to increase the eligibility to a full year because they're worried about increasing costs by essentially doubling the enrollment. They know that this eligibility problem works to their and the patients' advantage. Also, with patients coming and going all the time and using a lot of services, we're stuck with a system where the patient doesn't stay in the system long enough. You can't recoup your losses like you can in a commercial plan."

"I thought you would find this table interesting. Just to give you an idea of how our managed Medicaid compared to our commercial experience for some key indicators," Josh said as he handed out the table (see Table 5–1).

"I pulled this together last night. You can see the differences in growth rates, disenrollment rates, late enrollees, retroactivity, and physician switches between commercial and managed Medicaid."

"You can see that our commercial HMO growth is around 5 percent, while our Medicaid growth is nearly 150 percent! We picked up a huge number of enrollees—sick enrollees I might add—when most other practices around opted out of the Medicaid plans. We became one of only a few 'players.'"

"The 'disenrollment rate' shows how many members leave the plan—mostly because of eligibility issues. In our commercial HMOs, there is very little disenrollment, around one-half of one percent. Even if an employer changes plans, we usually retain the member in our practice because we're in all of them. But with Medicaid, nearly one-third of our members disenroll sometime during the year. They come and go and come and go because of the short eligibility requirements.

"'Retroactive enrollment' shows how many members come into our practice after their eligibility date. You can see that about 4 percent of

Table 5–1 Comparison between Medicaid and Commercial HMO Indicators

Indicator	Commercial HMO	Medicaid HMO
Growth Rate	5% increase	150% increase
Disenrollment Rate	.5%	30%
Retroactive Enrollment	4%	35%
Physician "Switches"	.5%	15%

commercial members come on retroactively, but with Medicaid, you have nearly a third again!"

"Last, 'physician switches' represents the percentage of members' switching PCPs. Commercial members are pretty stable at less than one-half of one percent, but the Medicaid members switch docs a whole bunch more! This has to do with the 'freedom of choice' requirements of the Medicaid program and the 30-day allowance of the State."

"What this means, everyone, is that in the commercial population, we have a more or less stable group. We know for the most part who they are and if they're eligible or not. We can handle this group. However, the Medicaid population is a moving target—it's tough to draw a bead on them because they're always in and out and back in again. And even when they're in, they switch docs so continuity of care, compliance with treatment plans, etc. are constant problems."

Al interjected, "And remember, last year the State expanded coverage. They went from traditional Medicaid families, AFDC—usually single moms with one or more children—to include general assistance, you know, those who qualify for standard Medicaid and fall below federal poverty guidelines, the elderly, and the disabled. So not only do we have the issues Josh described in this table, we also have whole new classes of members, with unique health care needs!"

Josh took the opening, "And remember, they have a *single* capitation rate for all classes of eligible folks. Now isn't that insane! They pay the same rate for the elderly or the disabled as for the traditional Medicaid person. They tell us that it is a 'blended' cap rate, and that it takes different utilization rates into account. But the rate is less than most of our commercial cap rates. We need an age and sex capitation rate for each category of

Medicaid member: AFDC, elderly, disabled. Then we would be in better shape."

"Can providers expect to break even seeing these kinds of patients?" asked Dr. Kaplan.

"Under the current circumstances, clearly no," replied Josh.

"Wait a minute, Josh," said Al. "Didn't they sell this plan to us as a way for us to at least cover our costs?"

"That's what they said, but clearly it isn't turning out that way," replied Josh. "The hospitals have been doing pretty well though. Their bad debt and charity care dried up when more people got coverage. They're not capped and were able to negotiate half-decent rates. A lot of the hospitals have actually benefited from managed Medicaid in the State. Maybe that's who they were talking about."

"It seems to me that whoever holds the risk loses in an *underfunded* managed Medicaid program," said Dr. Kaplan. "If the State keeps the risk, they lose. If the plans keep the risk and pay us fee-for-service, the plans lose. If the providers accept the risk, we lose."

"Exactly!" said Josh. "When 'capitation' is little more than a thinly disguised legislative appropriation, it becomes a zero-sum game, plain and simple. When there's not enough money in the system, the one who's holding the risk. . .loses. And right now, that's us."

"Even some of the Medicaid MCOs are throwing in the towel," said Al. "They're getting out of the program, citing big losses. The State is talking about putting more money into the system, but it's too late for two or three plans. They're going under."

No one spoke, but everyone in the room was thinking the same thought. Would Healthtron be joining them?

"That raises some interesting issues," said Dr. Kaplan. "With fewer plans remaining, we have more patients over fewer plans, so our ability to manage this mess becomes even more critical."

"It's nearly impossible to manage 'this mess' as it's now structured," said Al. "We have several strikes already against us—the eligibility mess, the capitation rate problems, the lack of State monitoring, the arbitration problems, and we haven't really talked about the 'due process' issues."

"Tell us about them, Al," Dr. Kaplan said.

"Well, under long-established legal principles, Medicaid recipients, even those enrolled in managed care, are guaranteed 'due process' rights under the U.S. Constitution. At a minimum, due process requires that a Medicaid recipient receives written notice and an opportunity for a timely hearing before an impartial decision maker before any service is reduced, denied, or delayed. MCOs that violate these due process rights risk violating federal law, so they don't control utilization nearly as tightly as they do on a commercial line of business. We've seen case after case where the State's Appeal Board has overturned the MCO's utilization management decisions. In fact, nearly 90 percent of the time the decisions are overturned, and the services are required to be delivered to the patient. This is maybe better care, I don't know, but it sure creates an incentive for the MCOs to slack off, especially if they have down-streamed significant portions of the risk to us providers. If they kept the risk, they're getting killed with the additional administrative overhead of all the appeals and hearings as well as then providing the care anyway. This is one reason some of the plans are packing up and going home.

"Yes, for most plans we're just seeing 'managed care' is managing access to care and managing provider reimbursement," said Al.

"You're right, Al," said Josh. "I don't care if it's a Wall Street MCO or a provider-sponsored HMO, the imperative is short-term profits. It's their mantra—short-term profits, short-term profits—so no one is really thinking long term. Investors want results immediately, and provider-sponsored plans keep sinking capital into these things and losing their shirts so everyone is under extreme pressure to do two things—manage access to care and manage provider reimbursement through risk shifting.

"I guess that's why they're not paying our claims on time," said Dr. Kaplan.

"That's true," explained Josh. "We've already discussed the avalanche of members dumped onto the plans—200,000 people overnight! That's a whole city, for crying out loud! They have to find these Medicaid people, get them to complete enrollment forms, including the selection of a PCP, and load them into their systems. Like I said before, this is not an easy population to find, much less enroll effectively. In many cases, the old Medicaid systems couldn't give the data to the MCOs without a lot of programming. Then the people start using three or four times the health care resources that a commercial population uses, and all these claims start hitting their system.

"Meanwhile, they've staffed their claims department with commercial ratios of staff instead of the greater number of Medicaid claims processors needed, either because they didn't know any better or because they were so focused on short-term profits. They have to hire and train all those bodies—enough for 200,000 members! Not even the Blues can swallow that many members without having to hire and train a bunch of people off the street. And a lot of these people have never paid claims before—they just saw an ad in the paper and needed a job. So they have a big learning curve, including medical terminology, coordination of benefits, subrogation, HCFA 1500 data elements, CPT codes, ICD codes, the claims processing system, etc.

"Then everyone has to learn the new claims processing system because the old one wouldn't do, and the systems guys aren't able to get it working correctly right away. So by the time the MCO gets its act together, it's already six to nine months behind in claims. They have paper coming out their ears, because they haven't figured out how to get the electronic claims submission working yet. We providers are all screaming since our cash flow is drying up. So we resubmit and resubmit and resubmit and call and call and call. So now there's more paper with all the resubmissions and the phones are so tied up that no one can get through. We scream at the State. The State screams at the MCOs. The MCOs promise to catch up. But they can't. Their paid claims and IBNR figures go through the roof, so their books are a disaster. Everyone's miserable.

"If it was a commercial population, we would bill the patient—even if the contract says we can't, just to get them to scream at the health plan. But with Medicaid, we can't do that because these people won't scream at the health plan.

"To top everything off, they tell us there is a 60-day time limit for filing claims, so any claims that we got to them past the 60-day filing limit are denied contractually. Granted, we should be able to get our claims out in 60 days, under normal circumstances—but these are not normal circumstances! There are always AR problems, especially with eligibility information, lack of ID cards, unsigned forms, data entry, etc. that mess us up. So on Day 61 we find out we've been billing the wrong MCO for the past two months, and we're out of luck. Oh, sure, we can tell them that we're sorry, that there was a miscommunication. They'll smile and say, 'Sorry. We can't pay that claim.'"

The room was quiet. Everyone knew Josh was right. They had seen it firsthand. "Thank you, Josh," said Dr. Kaplan. Nothing more needed to be said.

"Monica, what's happening with pharmacy costs?" asked Dr. Kaplan. Monica was in charge of tracking pharmacy costs for the practice. "Pharmacy is killing us." It was unusual for Monica to be so blunt, but Josh's influence was spreading. "We're budgeted at $2.89 per member per month, and we're running at $7.05 per member per month. And it's climbing at 70 percent per year."

"Why?" asked Dr. Kaplan.

"The original cap rate was way off and after they shifted the risk of the pharmacy to the providers, they opened up the formulary. So our docs love it, but we're losing our shirts."

"Can you talk to the physicians," asked Dr. Kaplan, "and ask them to voluntarily limit their use of prescriptions?"

Monica winced. "I could, but I know what I'll hear. 'I'm trained to get the best medical results. I need that drug to heal my patient. I'm not going to compromise my care just to save a buck. My professional ethics are not for sale.'"

Josh interjected, "Our docs are paid a salary, and so they have every incentive to use what they feel is the best drug for the job and to not worry about the cost."

"Unless we go out of business or lay some off," corrected Dr. Kaplan.

Josh did not back down. "True. But my point is that our internal incentive systems are messed up. We took on substantial health care risk without the systems or incentives in place to change behavior. We're still doing things 'the way we've always done them.' We should have installed that contact capitation software when we had the chance last year. You remember that manic little consultant that told us how to 'contact capitate' everyone. What was his name? Started with a C, I think. . .anyway, our infrastructure just wasn't ready for this deal."

Dr. Kaplan and everyone else in the room knew he was right. They had gotten into a bad deal—accepting too much risk—and hadn't been prepared to manage it.

"You're right, Josh," said Al, "but it's not like we haven't been trying. We've added three new medical records people, a full-time preauthorization reviewer, I don't know how many people in Accounts Receivable, and another front desk person to check eligibility as best we can. The additional administrative burden of managed Medicaid is incredible for a practice like ours—we have to deal with utilization management, additional front desk requirements, outcomes, patient satisfaction surveys, HEDIS requirements, performance measures—stuff like that."

"Yes, Al," replied Josh, " those things are all great, but we haven't invested in systems—like a new AR system that can handle managed care and capitation more effectively, or a contact capitation system in order to pay our people using sane incentives, or even training our administrative and medical people on managed care principles or on the risks we've taken on in this deal. It's no wonder that we're doing things 'the way we've always done them'. . .no one knows that things are different except us."

"Okay," said Dr. Kaplan, "what else?"

Monica began, "Well, we're having a serious problem with access to specialists. The Medicaid network has so few specialists that we can't find anyone to refer our very sick patient to. When we can find someone, they're often too far away for the patient to travel to. So our docs and mid-levels spend hours on the phone trying to get a specialist to accept someone, and then more hours on the phone to the MCOs trying to convince them to approve an out-of-network referral."

Al interjected, "As primary care docs, this leaves us with a huge potential liability since we're the ones treating the patient, and we have little or no specialist support. We can't meet the needs of the patient; we can't abandon the patient; if anything goes wrong, we're in trouble." Monica agreed.

Al continued, "Another related problem to this is just the whole 'discontinuity of care.' I worry about it. Patients are batted back and forth among MCOs; the Behavioral Health Organizations were created when the State carved out mental health and alcohol and drug so we have to deal with them; patients are noncompliant with treatment plans much of the time; we can never reach people by phone. . .I don't know, it just seems like we have a very fragmented health care system with a lot of people with very serious conditions not complying with treatment and with no access to specialists. Some patients are belligerent; a dozen family members all show up with one patient and clog the waiting rooms; care is in disarray. Some are drug seekers; some aren't. Many patients can't establish a positive PCP relationship, or vice versa, so they come and go and switch docs. There is little continuity of care. It's a recipe for a medical disaster, and I don't think any of us have addressed the whole liability risks we're running each day we're open."

"Welfare reform is increasing our medical risk, too," said Josh.

"How's that?" asked Dr. Kaplan.

"As we all know, welfare reform is shrinking the welfare rolls. People who can work, who can contribute in some way, are coming off the rolls and out of Medicaid. Who do you think is left?"

"Sicker patients," replied Dr. Kaplan.

"That's right!" said Josh. "Sicker patients for whom we're capitated. Our risk just went up again."

"I hate to bring this up," said Dr. Kaplan, "but what about the MCO's management information systems and the whole Y2K problem?"

"Well," Josh said, "our systems are up to date and can handle the Year 2000, so there's no problem there. In fact, we've done an entire Y2K audit of all our computers, medical equipment, phone systems, the works. And we're okay. But we just got a letter from our major MCO saying that their systems are not Y2K compliant, and that we should, and I quote, 'prepare for some minor disruptions of claims and utilization management systems.'"

"What does that mean?" asked Dr. Kaplan.

"We don't know," replied Josh. "but it is indicative of the MCOs nearly always being behind the eight ball when it comes to MIS. They've had a tough time the last few years with premiums being low and their medical and administrative costs going through the roof, so they've slacked off on investing in infrastructure improvements, including Y2K, until it's too late. The Y2K problem is going to hurt some of these guys I'm afraid."

"Okay," said Dr. Kaplan, "have we exhausted all the problems?"

She looked around the room and saw the frustration and anxiety on everyone's face. She knew she had a good team in place and was now ready to move them from problem-focused thinking to solution-focused thinking.

Dr. Kaplan pulled out her notes.

"First of all, I want to thank each of you for the hard work you're doing. I'm proud of each of you. Our financial situation is shaky, but we're on solid ground with the talents and commitment of each of you. So let's develop a plan on how we're going to fix this mess," she said. "Okay, here are a few ideas I've had while we've talked. Feel free to add to them as I go down the list," Dr. Kaplan said. "Here's my five-point plan to turn things around:

Strategy #1: Renegotiate our managed Medicaid contracts with the following points in mind:

- Renegotiate the capitation rates. We need age, sex, and Medicaid category cap rates, *not* a blended rate. We need to know our costs per member per month by age, sex, and Medicaid category. We also need to go to the State Insurance Department and get our hands on the MCOs' rate filings. As you all know, every state requires that rates be filed. This will help us with unit cost and utilization assumptions.

- Get procedure codes in writing. We need to know exactly, by procedure code, what we're at risk for. This applies to our existing contract as well as our newly negotiated one.
- Change the arbitration language. Al, use the language that you told us about, requiring the use of the AAA procedures. That will clear up a lot of these problems.
- Shed unmanageable risk. As a matter of policy, we need to get rid of any risk that we can't manage. I'm thinking about pharmacy especially and also inpatient risk.

Strategy #2: Obtain accurate, timely eligibility files. Many of our receivable problems stem directly from our lack of eligibility information.

- Review our contract to see what the MCO is required to provide us in terms of eligibility information.
- Investigate other sources of eligibility information, such as State Medicaid eligibility files, commercial tracking products and Internet files.
- Get a better handle on the retroactivity issue. We need a strategy to not only understand retroactive effective dates, but also a strategy to work with hospitals to inform us when a potential patient of ours is admitted so we can handle the case from the start.

Strategy #3: Improve our own internal infrastructure to better manage the changes we're facing.

- Train each and every staff member on managed Medicaid—how it works, our incentives, our disincentives, our contracts, etc. I know this will take some time to do right, but we have no choice. Only if everyone knows what's going on, will we be able to work together.
- Submit each claim accurately within 60 days. Look, we can't afford to miss claim submission deadlines on top of everything else. This is just

one of the challenges when we're running in a mixed capitation and fee-for-service system. We need a clear strategy on how we're going to increase cash flow through more effective and accurate claims submissions.

- Install contact capitation. One of our problems is that as an organization, we've been slow to change over to better technology that aligns financial incentives. We need to pay our physicians differently, and contact capitation is the best way I know to fairly pay people working in a capitated environment based on contacts. We also need to build in incentives for administrative people, both front desk and back office people, to share in improved systems and doing things right.

- Review and change our internal policies and procedures. We need to make a lot of changes in the way we treat patients based on the new realities. For example, we've been reluctant to embrace clinical protocols or pathways. Maybe we need to rethink the way we treat patients, especially in a world that is much more fragmented and has less access to specialty care.

- Establish an Internal Review Committee for all managed care contracts. Look, we did the best we knew how on the old contract, but now we're smarter and know what to look for and what to look out for. We need to put the best minds in the company to work reviewing and negotiating these contracts. If we can't live with the contract and the MCO says, 'Take it or leave it,' we need this group to make the recommendation. The days of rolling over on contracts are over. We see where that strategy has gotten us.

- Improve our own internal precertification procedures. I'm not sure we do a very good job here, so let's look into it and make sure our front desk people know what to do so our back office people can collect.

Strategy #4: Conduct member education. I know your concerns about noncompliance, PCP relationships, etc., but I also know that if we work at better communication and education of our members, we'll reap dividends.

- Develop a member education and training package that's sensitive to time, reading levels, culture, language, and whatever else we think is important. Talk about prevention, our expectations for care, managed care, ID cards, etc. Help our members understand, and we'll have fewer problems. I think we'll even see improved quality of care and outcomes.

Strategy #5: Implement a strong lobbying effort directed at our State Medical Association, the State Medicaid officials, our elected officials, and HCFA. Since Josh made the point so clearly that there is a lot of politics in managed Medicaid, we need to pull those strings.

- We need to get the word out that there are many problems with the system, and that we're getting killed.
- Tell them we need more and better State oversight of the program in very specific areas like claims, Y2K, reimbursement rates, contracting, and network adequacy (especially specialists).
- We need to make sure that we communicate the importance of treating primary care providers right, or the whole managed Medicaid program will come crashing down when we all pull out.
- Investigate Section 1902 of the Federal Code. We've said that this section is generally not waived in State waivers, and it really protects providers. We need to understand it better and see how we can use it to our advantage. Providers in other states have challenged the State in Federal Court based on this section. We need some good legal advice here.
- Beat the EPSDT drum. No state is doing a very good job with EPSDT for kids. We're seeing only 15 percent of eligible Medicaid kids getting the screenings and care they're entitled to. Our legislators need to know that EPSDT is important for our kids and that managed care is hurting it and us."

Dr. Kaplan asked, "Any questions or discussion?"

Her colleagues looked around at each other. They were visibly relieved that they had a plan. "It makes a lot of sense," said Josh.

"I like it," said Al. "I think it captures solutions to what we discussed. I'm sure it will evolve as we proceed, but it's a good start in the right direction."

Monica nodded agreement.

"Good," said Dr. Kaplan. "I'll assign responsibilities and timelines and get everything out to you in writing by tomorrow. We'll have a progress meeting every Monday at 7 AM. Thank you."

They left the room silently. They realized that they were facing perhaps the greatest challenge of their health care careers, and all left with a greater appreciation of the human, technological, medical, legal, economic, and political complexities they needed to face in order to survive, and hopefully thrive, in the new world of managed Medicaid.

REFERENCES

1. S. Rogers, "Why Are HCFA Waivers Necessary?" *The Key* 3, No. 3 (Fall-Winter 1996).
2. American Arbitration Association. "Commercial Arbitration Rules, as Amended and Effective on July 1, 1996." http://www.adr.org (1997).
3. Ibid.
4. Social Security Act, §1902(a)(30)(A), 42 U.S.C. §1396a(a)(30)(A).

SUGGESTED READINGS

Gold, M. et al. 1996. Medicaid Managed Care: Lessons from Five States. *Health Affairs* 15, No. 3: 153–160.

Rogers, S. 1996. Why are HCFA Waivers Necessary? *The Key* 3, no: 3.

Commercial Arbitration Rules, as Amended and Effective on July 1, 1996. 1997. *American Arbitration Association.* www.adr.org.

CHAPTER 6

Avoiding "Surprises" in Specialty Capitation

Clifford R. Frank, MHSA

INTRODUCTION

As HMO payers and providers look for new ways to conduct their affairs, specialty capitations are becoming more common. This chapter identifies key issues and problems that occur when developing a specialty capitation program. This analysis is based on the actual experience of several programs and will help providers and their advisors anticipate and/ or avoid similar design and operational problems.

Understanding the range of motivations for building a specialty capitation program is important because several downstream decisions are affected by the underlying reasons for seeking this sort of arrangement in the first place. For a payer, the reasons may be to control excessive utilization, to steer patients to a higher quality program, to enhance marketability of the payer, and many other possibilities. For providers, specialty capitation may be simply a move to protect existing market share, to gain leverage over a segment of the business, or to enter new markets to expand the reach of the provider's specialty program. In any case, new business or old, capitation is a new way of doing business, fraught with potential pitfalls and unpleasant surprises.

FIRST STEPS

Sorting out the questions to answer in developing a specialty capitation arrangement is no small trick. The logical flow that seems to work best is from covered services to provider network design, to payment rates and operational problems, and data reporting needs. What, who, how, how much, and what's happening?

What Is Covered?

In negotiating a specialty capitation, providers must have a thorough understanding of what is included, how such services and patients are to be identified, and what services are specifically carved out or excluded from the capitation. Services included in a specialty capitation can vary depending upon the needs of the payer, the capabilities of the provider, and the geographic coverage requirements imposed by the market.

In identifying services to be covered, here are the major issues:

- Is the capitation for professional services only, or does the capitation also include facility inpatient and/or outpatient costs?

Issue A: If the capitation is a global one that includes both hospital and physician costs, the implementation and operational systems must be more carefully thought through.

Explanation: In a global capitation, many hospital operational procedures can inadvertently impact the capitation pool. Non-capitated physicians on emergency room call schedules, non-capitated physicians reading EKGs, duplication of testing at the hospital and physician offices, consultation requests from inpatient nursing units to non-capitated physicians, and other potential complications can drain the professional pool of capitated funds quickly.

Issue B: If the specialty capitation is a global specialty capitation (it includes both clinical services and institutional costs), how are patients restricted to just the participating physicians and facilities, especially in emergent or urgent situations?

Explanation: Just because an HMO says all specialty services will be provided by a designated physician panel there is no guarantee that it will happen that way. The patient may be directed to the nearest emergency room that happens to not be a participating facility in the capitation program. HMO primary care physicians may refer the patient to the wrong specialist. The emergency room can call in the wrong specialist internists and family practice physicians can provide some specialty services and may get called in on a case, instead of the capitated specialist. Who pays, who is at risk?

- Are all clinical services included in the specialty capitation—including those specialty services provided by general internists and family practitioners?

Issue: If all services are included, how does the HMO propose to restrict the provider panel to specialists, and who pays for specialty services provided by other physicians?

Explanation: The problems raised by this issue are extensive and complicated. First, internists and family practitioners often refer to specialists. But they also perform some of these services themselves. If the HMO is capitating a group of cardiologists for cardiology services, then who tells the other physicians that they must now not treat those patients they used to treat for that HMO? If the cardiologists tell the internists and family practitioners, the cardiologists run the risk of seriously antagonizing their primary referral base. If the hospital imposes those restrictions, the hospital runs a similar risk. If the HMO imposes the restriction that all cardiology is now handled only by the cardiology capitation group, then the HMO runs the risk of seriously alienating its primary care base. These primary care physicians take great pride in their ability to treat many of their patients involved with HMOs. To deny them access to those patients is to insult their professional capabilities. But to not restrict the provision of cardiology services to those capitated cardiologists creates the potential for the HMO to pay for the same service twice (once to the primary care physician and again to the cardiologist through the specialty capitation). The alternative is to have those costs built into the capitation rate, and deduct the cost of services provided by the internists and family practitioners from the cardiologists' capitation. This situation arises in most medical specialty subcapitation arrangements.

- How are specialty cases to be identified as ones that are covered under the global specialty capitation?

Issue: Not all services a specialist performs may be unique to that specialty. Not all medical services initially thought to be cardiac remain so, e.g., the suspected heart attack that turns out to be indigestion. How are these services to be accounted for under a capitated specialty program?

Explanation: For a specialty global capitation program that includes hospital claims, the primary discharge diagnosis should govern whether the services are capitated or not. If this primary discharge diagnosis from an inpatient stay is cardiac related, then it falls under the cardiac capitation. If the diagnosis upon discharge is something else, then even though the cardiologists provided the professional services, the inpatient facility fee should be paid outside the capitation. This decision rule resolves the situation where the heart attack turned out to be indigestion.

For professional services provided by physicians, the HMO will probably want to say that anything the capitated specialist does is included in the capitation. This simplifies immeasurably the administration of the program. However, this also means that any specialist who performs other services will find them capitated, and the compensation arrangement may not be satisfactory as a result. For the HMO, the priority is making sure it does not pay for a service twice—once under capitation and again as fee-for-service. The resulting delineation of responsibilities for medical providers may not neatly fit with existing practice arrangements and may impact the decision about which practitioners participate.

- What services are generally excluded from a specialty capitation program?

Issue: Not all specialty networks cover all services for all patients. Certain exclusions may need to be negotiated to avoid taking undue risk.

Explanation: Heart transplants, pediatric specialty services or congenital conditions, and other specialized procedures may be excluded or "carved out" of the capitation. If such exclusions are negotiated, care associated with the patient prior to the transplant may also be carved out if clear diagnoses or procedural designations can be identified. Other common exclusions are out-of-area emergency care, and sometimes in-area emergencies at non-capitated facilities can also be excluded.

- How are emergencies handled in a specialty capitation program?

Issue: Specialty emergencies often do not allow a network physician or network facility to treat the patient even if the illness occurs while the patient is in the HMO's service area. What "fair" arrangements can be negotiated to handle this costly risk?

Explanation: First, let's distinguish between two types of emergencies: in-area and out-of-area. Most capitation agreements exclude or carve out out-of-area costs because the situation is completely outside the control of the local network. Most HMOs budget separately for out-of-area emergency claims anyway, so this exclusion should not be hard to negotiate.

However, in-area emergencies are another matter. Many HMOs believe that emergency services are handled very divergently by different treating physicians. Two similar cases may have costs that are wildly different for no other reason than the physician's treatment choices. That's the HMO's motivation for wanting to capitate specialty services in the first place. The HMOs will most likely want to stick the in-area emergencies into the specialty capitation. That means that the costs associated with emergencies treated by physicians other than those in the capitated network will be deducted from the capitation payment to the specialty network. Clearly, such deductions could adversely affect the financial performance of the capitation for participating specialists.

Capitated specialists would most likely prefer to exclude in-area emergencies not treated at their primary facilities to limit the risk and financial exposure from non-contracting specialists. The practical alternatives are these:

1. Make sure that specialists at each hospital are included in the capitated network,
2. Limit the time or dollar amount in other facilities for which the capitated network will be responsible, or
3. Accept risk only when the patients are transferred to network facilities and the care of network specialists.

In a large metropolitan area, including specialists at all hospitals is simply not practical and will so dilute the focus of the network as to ensure everyone's financial demise in the capitation program. Limiting exposure by time or dollars makes some sense and can be successfully negotiated. The rationale is that if the patient can be transferred in two days, then effective clinical intervention by the capitated network can have beneficial effects for both the network and the HMO. However, if the patient cannot be stabilized in two days, then the patient is probably very ill, and the case is going to be very expensive. The HMO has its own large case management systems that will likely work as well as the network's do for large cases. The alternative of accepting risk only when the patients arrive at contracting facilities is certainly the easiest to manage and understand.

- What is a reasonable capitation rate, and what is it based upon?

It depends, it depends, it depends . . . on covered services, covered populations, and payment rate requirements of participating providers.

Which Providers Are in the Specialty Network?

- Who determines who is included in the specialty capitation network?

Issue: Who picks the providers? Does the HMO pick? Does a network just "come together?" Do certain physicians or physician groups pick? Does the hospital organize the network?

Explanation: Who picks, and on what basis, is an extremely sensitive and volatile question. HMOs like to pick because they think it is their job to do so. However, they can make poor choices such as splitting a call group, picking junior partners in a practice while excluding the senior physicians, or choosing physicians to please the HMO's major customers rather than choosing efficient physicians. On the other hand, if physicians simply gravitate toward each other, selections can result that have more to do with who gets along, rather than who is most efficient. If the hospital tries to organize the network, everyone will be mad because of the perceptions that the hospital is playing favorites—regardless of the clinical criteria used. There is no quick or easy way to organize the network that ensures the most efficient physicians are included and that peace reigns within the walls of the hospital.

Because the entire process is fraught will pitfalls, aggressive specialty groups can make headway by moving rapidly and quietly in direct negotiation with HMOs. If an HMO is approached with a reasonable-looking specialty network panel, their inclination will be to consider it, rather than simply opening up the process to all comers. An important consideration for HMOs is whether members of the proposed specialty network already contract with the HMO. If yes, the decision the HMO faces is less difficult—a decision to shrink the network in a particular specialty. If the specialists do not currently contract with the HMO, the decision is much more difficult. The HMO may not have good data on the network's practice patterns and economic performance. The HMO may be reluctant to face the wrath of its customers as it contemplates switching large numbers of patients from one specialty panel to another. The HMO may not be comfortable with the specialty network's track record for working through administrative issues. These hurdles make turning HMO specialty care over to a new network very risky for the HMO and not very attractive. This means that most specialty capitations will emerge as slimmed down panels from existing participants until a specialty market leader is firmly established.

- What factors should be considered when selecting physicians to participate in the specialty capitation program?

Issue: Choosing partners in a venture is always difficult. Forming a specialty network is no exception. Developing a rational basis for physician selection is important to avoid adding to conflicts that already exist within the medical staff.

Explanation: Having objective, measurable criteria for inclusion would be the ideal manner for choosing physicians. However, such criteria and measurements are often lacking beyond the most basic elements such as board certification, malpractice experience, hospital disciplinary actions, and related indicators. Ideally, the specialty network needs cost-effective practitioners, with accessible schedules, experienced in working with groups of physicians, who can adapt to the requirements of practicing under a capitated program. Measuring physician resource utilization by type of case, severity adjusted if possible, would be a starting point. Understanding surgical frequencies, major diagnostic test frequencies, and other major occurrences are important as well. Capitation programs don't usually get into trouble because the surgeons or clinicians want too much per case. The problem often is that they perform too many procedures as compared to the budgeted amount built into the capitation. The network must choose physicians who can practice to the requirements of the program and feel comfortable in doing so. If the medical leadership of the network is going to have to fight the network physicians each step of the way, then there is something fundamentally wrong.

Another dimension to physician selection is the track record each physician has with the managed care insurance companies. If a particular specialist has been removed from panels for being too difficult or for excessive utilization, then including that physician in the capitation network may adversely affect the network's ability to contract with managed care payers. Most insurance companies now know which physicians they don't want. If the network includes physicians who are otherwise not viewed favorably by the customer (the insurance companies), the network is possibly compromised from the start.

How Do We Get Paid?

• How is the money split among the participating providers?

Issue: There are lots of ways to split the money. For a population of 40,000 enrollees with a cardiology global capitation of $3.60 per member per month ($1.20 physician, $2.40 hospital) the pot is $144,000 per month. How should these funds be distributed?

Explanation: Using cardiology as an example, inside a cardiology capitation should be a number of subcapitations. The object is to get as far away from fee-for-service thinking as possible, while maintaining fairness among the physicians doing the work. The cardiology capitation should be split into several pools—hospital, clinical, diagnostic, surgical, emergency. The hospital risk is the easiest to segregate. In the example above, of the $3.60 per member per month, $2.40 was reserved for hospital expenses, or $96,000 per month. That money should be set aside to cover hospital costs including testing, rehab, and emergency room costs at participating hospitals. If testing is going to be performed in physician offices, then a certain capitation amount ($.05–$.08 for example) should be transferred from the hospital pool to the physicians at the front end of the process.

Within the capitation pool, or within the subcapitation pools, funds still need to be allocated to practitioners serving their patients. Funds can be split evenly among all participants with the hope that the work also splits the same way. Or a more reliable allocation method can be used. Often a fee schedule is used to distribute funds, with monies being withheld to cover reserves, out-of-network liabilities, and claims incurred by a provider, but not yet received (IBNR). The trick here is to set the fee schedule right. Fee schedules assume a budgeted level of utilization because the number of service times the fee schedule must be less than or equal to the money in the pool each month. Otherwise, the fee schedule ends up consuming more funds than are available, and a deficit results. Deficits are disastrous because physicians hate to pay money back to a pool because somebody else in the network may have overutilized.

Rather than using a fixed fee schedule, a better method is to use one that floats—and balances automatically to the money available in the monthly pool. It works like this: Take a relative value scale, like the Resource Based Relative Value Scale (RBRVS). Tally the total claims turned in from a month of services and determine the total number of relative value points consumed—for example, 1,600 relative value points. Then divide the total number of relative value points into the related capitation pool, $1.20 per member per month (pmpm) times 40,000 members, or $48,000. Each point would be worth $30 that month. If a particular physician performed 205 points, he or she would receive a check that month for $6,150. The following month, if only 1,200 relative value points were consumed, each point would be worth $40, assuming the enrollment stayed constant. By having the point value, or conversion factor, float the pool always balances to the money available and never ends in deficit.

One quirk with the relative value scale method of disbursement is that the medical and surgical relative values on some relative value scales are quite different. This may necessitate an algebraic conversion of the relative value scale to standardize the conversion factors.

Another way to pay specialists inside a capitation pool is based on the number of active patients that a specialist is treating. This method, called contact capitation, pays each specialist his or her pro rata share of the capitation pool each month based upon the number of unique individual patients under treatment instead of using production of procedures to drive revenue. The contact capitation method pays physicians to treat each patient and divides funds within the specialty capitation pool based on patients, not procedures.

What Operational Problems Should We Anticipate?

- How do we differentiate capitated cases from others?

Issue: Managing capitated specialty cases early in the treatment cycle is important if utilization is going to be effectively controlled. Identifying capitated patients is an important, but difficult, patient registration function.

Explanation: Early identification and management of specialty capitation patients is key to the financial success of the program. Yet, these patients will not usually have an identification card specifically for this program. Their ID card will simply read "ABC HMO" and the patient registration people have to remember this. HMO is a capitation contract. Early identification of capitated cases allows for more active medical management by at-risk specialists, more aggressive case management, closer scrutiny of elective procedures, and routing of cases to the most efficient practitioner. Failure to identify capitated cases may mean that a non-network specialist, internist, or family practice physician spends time and resources caring for the patient to the detriment of capitated physicians.

- What happens if capitated physicians disagree about a course of treatment?

Issue: Physicians often do not agree about clinical decisions, but the physicians are not usually financially intertwined with each other. In a capitated system, medical judgments by one physician impact the financial outcome of others in the risk pool.

Explanation: Having a mechanism to resolve professional conflict is important to the success of the capitated program. Often a program medical director is empowered to settle both financial and clinical issues. Others use a medical committee. What's important is to have a mechanism to resolve professional disagreements, preserve quality, and monitor cost. Usually that means someone has to be explicitly in charge of those functions and empowered to make decisions stick.

- What happens if a non-network specialist is called by the emergency room or nursing personnel on the inpatient unit in error?

Issue: On-call schedules are often difficult for hospital personnel to manage, and building subgroups of capitated physicians makes the situation worse. In cases where a non-network physician takes a call, the source for payment for those services is an open question.

Explanation: The specialty capitation program probably includes emergency room coverage at contracting hospitals. If the ER or hospital unit manager makes a mistake and contacts the wrong specialist, that non-network specialist is still going to expect payment for his or her services. The non-network specialist will bill the HMO, the patient, the hospital, the ER group, the specialty network, or the insurance commissioner—but bills will definitely be sent. Such billings create the impression at the HMO that the hospital and the specialty network can't get their act together. The patient will complain about being billed to the HMO, and the problem for the specialty network doubles. Capitation programs are difficult enough to pull off without adding member relations problems to the mix. If this type of event occurs frequently, it could jeopardize the specialty capitation contract as a whole.

Some HMOs will pay the non-network specialist and deduct the payment from the network's next capitation payment. Others will forward the bill to the specialty network for approval and payment by the network. Some networks will, in turn, hand the bill to the hospital for payment since the hospital's staff called the wrong specialist. Systems to prevent misdirecting patients in the hospital are very important to the success of the program, and the hospital does bear some responsibility to ensure that the systems are in place and functioning. However, such administrative compliance cannot be assumed to happen; the network has to plan for it with contracting hospitals.

- Who reads the EKGs and how do they get paid?

Issue: Making sure that capitated physicians read EKGs on capitated patients is not always possible. But if charges are incurred by non-network physicians reading EKGs on capitated patients, who pays, and why?

Explanation: Reading EKGs is often included in the specialty capitation. Therefore, if a non-network cardiologist or internist reads the EKG of a capitated patient, that physician will expect to be compensated. Unless the hospital sets up a special procedure for separating out capitated patients' EKGs, expect chargebacks to the capitation pool for EKG reader fees. Most hospitals cannot segregate the capitated patients' EKGs and hold them for reading by a capitated physician. The EKG reader is usually on rotation among attending staff, and that physician takes all EKGs during a specific period.

- What special requirements does capitation place on the physician office staff?

Issue: Not all physician office staffs possess equal capabilities to perform important administrative functions. Solo offices have different patient booking procedures than do group practices. Communication with primary care physicians may vary among offices. Understanding differences in physician office style and accommodating them can be important to the success of the specialty capitation program.

Explanation: Each physician may require different tests or diagnostic procedures to work up a patient. Just as the network must develop a sense of reasonable clinical practices, so too must it develop administrative norms such as patient waiting time, access to care after hours, regular communication to the primary care physicians, and comfortable amenities of care. Staff who are sloppy, inattentive, rude, or inaccessible must be informed that their conduct is not in line with the expectations of the specialty capitation network. One shoddy office can pull down the whole network. This interconnectedness can pose major problems in two dimensions. First, many physicians and their office staff have never had to be accountable to anyone but themselves. Having an outsider, even if it is a physician colleague, inform them that their behavior, demeanor, or administrative systems are not up to par will be disconcerting at a minimum. The second dimension is an interpersonal one. Often in the smaller offices, the physician's spouse works in or runs the office. A challenge to the behavior, demeanor, or administrative systems of the physician office may be interpreted as a personal affront to the physician's spouse and may result in additional conflict within the specialty network.

- Isn't there a danger that capitated primary care physicians will "turf" questionable cases to capitated specialists?

Issue: Capitated primary care physicians face economic incentives to refer patients to specialists if their costs are not charged back to the primary care physician's incentive pools. The danger exists that primary care physicians may alter their scope of practice and refer cases to capitated specialists that PCPs previously would have managed themselves.

Explanation: "Turfing" patients to the capitated specialists is a very real possibility. The HMOs may say that they have referral protocols that require the patient to exhibit certain symptoms before a referral should be made. However, no capitated specialist is going to refuse a referral from a primary care physician for fear of potentially alienating that primary care physician on fee-for-service cases. "Turfing" can at least be monitored with the appropriate data system so that if one or two primary care physicians seem to be accounting for a disproportionate share of referrals, such a pattern can be identified. If such a pattern emerges, often the HMO medical director can become involved to counsel the offending primary care physicians. Certainly, budgeting a little extra in the clinical component of the capitation is wise in anticipating a mild referral surge.

- What is the collateral impact on medical staff relations at the hospital if only some of the specialists are included in the specialty capitation network?

Issue: Physicians who are not selected to participate in the specialty capitation program will likely be offended and view the hospital's involvement very suspiciously. Managing the emotional component of network selection decisions is key to hospital administration's survival and future credibility with the medical staff.

Explanation: The hospital has a very tough time getting involved in physician selection for capitated networks. This is best left to the HMO and its contracting specialists. Nonetheless, the hospital will be blamed by excluded physicians for either conspiring against them, or at least passively sitting by while others worked against these physicians' interests. The HMO needs to step forward and take responsibility for the decisions, and those decisions should have some rational basis—utilization-based, primary care physician preference, call group, specialty group, or other reasonable basis. Even if such a method is used, the emotional blow to many physicians of not being selected will far exceed any adverse financial impact. Physicians are generally used to being included, and this may be one of the few times when an entity or group has said, "No, thank you." For any physician who is excluded and is desirous of joining, the hospital's loyalty to that physician will be compared to that physician's loyalty to the hospital. The discussions can get quite heated, so having some other entity make the selections based on some measurable or defined criteria is important for everyone.

What Data Are We Going To Need?

- What decisions will we make with data?

Issue: Collecting data just to have them isn't usually productive in the long run. Data must be relevant to key decisions or collecting them ends up a waste of time and money.

Explanation: Data will be used to help with these decisions:

1. Who should get paid how much?
2. Who is overutilizing services?
3. Who may be underutilizing and jeopardizing quality of care?
4. How do we show employers and HMOs that we are doing a good job?
5. How do we know the deductions from the capitation are reasonable?

Claims data should be captured and routinely tabulated for each service provided by the specialty capitation network. Simply turning over a pot of money to a specialty group ensures that someone else will challenge the allocation of money down the road. Having data to support decisions is critical to establishing a sense of fairness and integrity to the process.

• Who should collect and manage the data?

Issue: Often the problem is not one of capabilities, but rather one of trust. If one entity is a provider and is also responsible for the data management, suspicions abound, particularly if things are going worse than initially projected.

Explanation: Some hospitals handle the capitation accounting for specialty networks, but every time the checks are "wrong," the capabilities and integrity of the hospital are called into question. Also, most hospitals lack the insurance knowledge and savvy necessary to administer a capitation program.

Those networks that have used outside capitation administrators report much higher satisfaction and less aggravation. The capitation administrator must understand setting up reserves for incurred-but-not-reported claims, in-area deductions, and other allocations. The capitation administrator must be able to generate meaningful physician profiles against group norms and outside utilization targets as well. The requirements go well beyond a clerk with a checkbook.

• What should we look for in a capitation administrator?

Issue: Many administrative entities will say they can handle capitation, but if they don't do it well, the network suffers far more than the administrator.

Explanation: A competent capitation administrator needs to be steeped in managed care knowledge and insurance operations. They must have the systems in place to generate meaningful financial and utilization reports. The specialty capitation network needs an administrator that can discern differences in treatment patterns, office procedures, and quirks in the data they are receiving from network providers in order to protect the integrity of the network as a whole. Many entities are available to simply write checks. But far fewer administrators can add valuable information to their analysis that can help the specialty capitation network save money over the long run.

- Who wrestles with the HMO over deductions from the capitation that look unfair or unwarranted?

Issue: Most capitation contracts allow the HMO to deduct monies from the capitation for certain occurrences such as emergency care. Sometimes the deductions may appear to be inappropriate and may require follow-up.

Explanation: The responsibility for the integrity of the funds in the specialty capitation should be the administrator's. If a deduction looks excessive or questionable, the administrator's job is to get the detailed information from the HMO about the claim, evaluate the information, and challenge the deduction if it seems inappropriate. If the administrator's challenge is not immediately successful, then the medical director of the network needs to get involved, but hopefully those situations seldom arise. Managing the deductions from the capitation is important because up to 10 percent or more of the capitation may be absorbed each month by chargebacks and other deductions.

- How do we determine which HMO members are eligible under the capitation program?

Issue: Having an HMO identification card is no guarantee that the member is still eligible. If the capitation is for members assigned just to certain primary care physicians or smaller geographic areas, eligibility cannot be determined just by looking at the member's identification card.

Explanation: The capitation administrator's job is to obtain from the HMOs and distribute member eligibility lists to provider offices. Also, claims for services provided to ineligible members must be returned to the provider so that the provider may bill the appropriate party.

- How does a capitation administrator compile normative data?

Issue: Having data for comparing individual physician performance is important in improving the overall performance of the specialty capitation network.

Explanation: The capitation administrator should be able to produce comparative data for the frequency of specific procedures. The problem in most comparisons is that providers are used to seeing comparisons among providers for ratios of procedures. What is far more meaningful is comparing the cath rate from provider to provider or network to network, and developing an understanding of how such variances occur. For example, one network may perform 8 cardiac caths per 1,000 people per year. Another network may do 5 cardiac caths per 1,000 people per year. Understanding that difference is critical to the financial success of the specialty network. Knowing what is reasonable on a utilization rate basis, and comparing the network's specific and aggregate performance to those norms can challenge a specialty capitation network's complacency long before deteriorating financial performance does.

CAUTIONS FOR THE FUTURE

Capitation for many specialties is here. For providers to survive under this new payment system, they must have the knowledge and capabilities of insurance companies. Managing risk, managing money, managing data, and managing quality all become intertwined and vital in capitation. Capitated providers who fail to invest in managing these functions are leaving themselves vulnerable. With capitation comes responsibility for managing risk. As in any enterprise, it is essential that you have the tools to manage successfully.

SUGGESTED READINGS

Stevens, L. 1999. Making Capitation Succeed in Your Practice Requires a Whole Different Mind-set. *American Medical News*, 26 July.

Capitation survey provides invaluable capitation data. 1997. *Healthcare Price, Cost & Utilization Benchmarks,* 16–28.

CHAPTER 7

Managing
Pharmaceutical Risk

*Steven R. Peskin, MD, MBA, FACP, Debi Reissman, Pharm.D.,
and Jonothan C. Tierce, C.Phil.*

THE SPIRALING OF DRUG COSTS

From 1996 through 1999, prescription drug program costs have escalated rapidly. The majority of health plans, plan sponsors, pharmacy benefit managers, and provider organizations that track pharmacy services costs have witnessed increases in the range of 15–20 percent in the period of 1996–1998, with this trend continuing into 1999. This rate of increase is substantially greater than any other segment of medical care costs.

The higher pharmacy trend rates are being driven largely by the following factors:

- new compounds, particularly biologics, that are substantially more expensive per dose or per course of therapy than existing products
- new categories of drugs or novel therapies that command a premium price and are not readily substitutable
- patient demand, in part driven by a surge in direct-to-consumer (DTC) advertising
- low, or relatively low, copayments or other out-of-pocket expenses
- improved diagnostic abilities and early identification of some conditions leading to earlier and increased prescribing of some drugs/ therapeutic classes

With respect to new compounds and novel therapies, there is a growing list of protein-based biologic/immune responses modifiers, which are typically high-cost injectables (greater than $1,000/mo) or high-cost infusion (greater than $2,000/dose) products. Additionally, higher cost new compounds are replacing less expensive compounds. There is also a trend toward an overall higher price point for new drugs. Lastly, there are growing numbers of so-called "lifestyle" drugs addressing the baby boomer generation's desire to appear young and maintain a more active lifestyle.

Fueling the demand for drug therapies, and particularly, for lifestyle drugs, is direct-to-consumer advertising. Additionally, a wealth of information is available on the Internet, on television and radio health programs—in addition to TV and radio advertising—and through other media channels.

In sharp contrast, other health services have ranged from being deflationary to increases of up to 8 percent. The dramatic increase in pharmacy costs has drawn tremendous attention from health plans and provider systems that bear financial risk for pharmacy services. Several health plan CEOs have singled out rising pharmacy costs as one of the most urgent issues that their organizations will need to address in order to improve health plan financial performance.

Although the price of older therapies has not been as important a factor, more recently price increases for some established therapies and for selected classes of multisource, i.e., generically available, products have experienced double-digit price increases. Reasons for this include a consolidation in manufacturers and availability of some multisource compounds from multiple to one or two generic manufacturers, shadow pricing, and a slower drop in price when products lose patent protection as compared to the period prior to 1995.

Except for copayments and other out-of-pocket expenses, health plans have limited ability to control the forces that are driving escalating pharmacy costs. Health plans are increasing copayments, and, in particular, are introducing three-tiered copayment structures that represent substantially higher patient cost sharing for the most expensive branded products. Additionally, health plans are now forcing the sharing of prescription program costs with contracted physicians or health care provider organizations by adding prescription costs to the hospital shared risk pool or medical services capitation rate.

PHARMACY BENEFIT DESIGNS

In general the outpatient prescription drug program offered through health plans provide coverage for oral and topical prescription agents. That being said, there is a multitude of subtle differences between benefit designs that can make it difficult to compare benefit costs and utilization statistics between health plans, especially when trying to determine cost projections when taking on pharmacy risk. Some of these differences include:

Self-Administered Injectables

Most health plans traditionally have not included injectable products under their prescription drug programs. This was because these agents generally required administration by health care personnel, and they were not stocked by retail pharmacies. However, with the introduction of products such as erythropoietin, interferons, etanercept, and others that are commonly self-administered, many health plans have begun covering these products under the pharmacy rather than the medical benefit. Health plans that include self-administered injectables in the pharmacy benefit have pharmacy program costs at least $1.00 per member per month (pmpm) higher than plans that do not include these agents. Some plans are reporting costs of as much as $3.00 pmpm for this class of agents.

Behavior Modification Products

Health plans may or may not cover products aimed at modifying patients' health behaviors, such as smoking cessation and diet pills, as part of the standard pharmacy benefit or supplementary benefit rider. Plans that cover these agents as part of their program typically add an additional $0.30 to $0.50 pmpm to the benefit.

Other Product Differences

Oral contraceptives, cosmetic treatments (such as Retin-A for wrinkles, antifungals for onychomycosis), infertility treatments, and diabetic testing materials are categories that vary in coverage among health plan prescription drug programs. Inclusion of these agents can add significant costs, from $0.30 pmpm for Retin-A or diabetic testing materials to $1.00 pmpm for oral contraceptives and infertility treatments.

Copayment Levels

Member copayments also vary among pharmacy benefit plan designs. Plans that have copayments that are at least $10 per prescription higher for brand agents as compared to generics typically yield higher use of generics resulting in lower overall costs versus plans that do not differ copayments between brand and generic agents. Similarly, plans that add a third copayment level for nonformulary agents find that their program costs and overall utilization patterns are lower versus plans that do not apply a copay differential for these nonpreferred agents. Each $1.00 change in copayment can alter overall costs by as much as $0.60 to $0.70 pmpm.

Quantity Limits

Plans that still allow a quantity of 100 units or a supply of more than 30 days to be dispensed through the retail pharmacy, without a compensatory increase in copayments, may have program costs $1.00 pmpm or more higher than other plans.

Formulary Controls

Controls such as prior authorization for nonformulary agents may be a significant deterrent to overprescribing of certain less cost-effective agents or those for which consumer demand may be fueling overutilization. As a result, plans with well-functioning prior authorization programs have better overall control over selected higher cost and discretionary agents resulting in pharmacy costs that may be up to $2.00 pmpm lower than other plans.

Rebates

Most health plans have been able to negotiate additional discounts from pharmaceutical manufacturers for the preferential use of their products. These discounts are calculated retrospectively based on the level of product use or market share of particular products as compared to their chief competitors. Payments are made after the plan demonstrates that the criteria for the "rebate" have been met. In general, product rebates do not exceed 15 percent of the product cost, are only available on brand products, and require the preferential use of the product as demonstrated by an increase in market share of the product as compared to other therapeutically equivalent options. Most plans find that the amount of rebate achievable is between 5 and 7 percent of the total drug program expenditure.

TAKING PHARMACY RISK

Risk programs for pharmaceuticals take many forms, from simple incentive/bonus systems to fully capitated programs. In general, risk program language is vague, generalized, and has historically not been an area of negotiation between health plans and provider groups or systems. Problems relate to provider organizations not understanding all of the issues involved in assuming pharmacy risk, not having the leverage to negotiate in order to provide reasonable financial protection to the group, or health plans being unwilling to negotiate.

Incentive/Bonus Programs

Bonus programs for pharmaceuticals generally focus on maintaining or improving key program indicators such as generic percentage, formulary compliance, and the number of prescriptions written per member per month. Meeting goals for these indicators would result in a bonus payment of X dollars pmpm. Rarely is there a penalty imposed if goals are not met. For successful programs, it is important to set the hurdles at levels only a few percentage points above current levels and look for improvement over the course of two to three years. For many providers, the goals are set too high compared to their current performance levels, making achievement of the goals virtually impossible within the annual contract cycle. As a result, many do not even try to meet the goals, as there is no financial penalty for nonachievement. This has caused health plans to move away from this type of arrangement and toward a program where cost overruns are also shared by the provider.

Shared Risk Programs

Similar to hospital withhold pools under shared medical risk agreements, shared pharmacy risk is also designed as a withhold pool and in most cases is actually attached to or becomes part of the overall hospital withhold program. This program has become the most popular form of pharmacy risk sharing as it provides for both positive and negative incentives related to prescribing. Under these programs, a budget is established for pharmacy expenses and then withheld into a pool rather than paid to the provider directly. All pharmacy expenses for patients enrolled with the provider organization are deducted from the pool with net deficits and surpluses split between the plan and provider. While some groups have been savvy enough to negotiate out of the program certain high cost agents, most groups have not asked the health plan to fully disclose what costs are assigned to the pool, resulting in surprise expenses at the end of the year.

Capitated and/or Full Risk Programs

A misnomer, capitated programs are in actuality usually full risk agreements. Rarely are the monies budgeted for pharmacy actually paid to the provider up front as in a capitation agreement. Typically, full risk agreements are designed just like the shared risk program except that deficits or credits from the withhold pool are the full responsibility of the provider rather than being shared with the health plan.

In order for physicians/provider organizations to manage pharmacy risk, the group or system needs to address the issues found in Exhibit 7–1. In addition, they should consider the evaluation criteria for pharmacy risk listed in Exhibit 7–2.

USE OF PHARMACOECONOMIC DATA

The development of the discipline of "pharmacoeconomics" has seen a dramatic expansion over the last decade. The amount of published literature containing cost-benefit or cost effectiveness of pharmaceuticals and other medical interventions has grown from but a few hundred citations in the early 1980s (see, for example, *Cost-Benefit and Cost-Effectiveness Analysis in Health Care*[1]) to literally thousands worldwide today. Able attempts to summarize the methods and apply them to the management and practice of health care include: *Principles of Pharmacoeconomics*[2] and *Quality of Life and Pharmacoeconomics in Clinical Trials*.[3] The published literature in most every disease and therapeutic area now contains a

Exhibit 7–1 Issues To Consider When Taking/Accepting Pharmacy Risk

Pharmacy Services Budget
Adequacy of the pharmacy services budget for the range of drugs covered under the contract (oral medications, self-administered injectables, outpatient intravenous medications, and high-cost therapies such as Ceredase™, Synagis™, or Enbrel™). Which agents, if any, should be reallocated to other catastrophic or stop-loss pools.

Track and Trend Costs
Ability to track and trend costs and utilization data (i.e., access to detailed information from the pharmacy benefit claim administrator employed by the health plan). How often will data be supplied and in what format.

Control over Formulary Management
Who has control over formulary decisions? How can group have input to formulary changes? What is group's ability to prescribe nonformulary agents?

Leadership
Leadership within the provider group that has experience with/commitment to working with prescribers on prudent, appropriate prescribing practices.

Resources
Internal staff or external resources competent in pharmacoeconomic analysis with the ability to effectively communicate findings and to facilitate physician/practitioner-led development of guidelines or step therapy protocols.

Assessment
Assessment of the interplay between pharmacy utilization/costs and overall medical care utilization/costs.

subliterature devoted to economic analyses. And, we are now beginning to see complete volumes devoted to the economics of a single disease area (see, for example, *Health Economics of Dementia*[4]).

Pharmacoeconomic methods are now available to managed care pharmacy managers to assist in the development of formulary policy, guidelines for prescriber and pharmacist practices, and drug benefit design. (See "The Application of Pharmacoeconomic in Managed Healthcare Set-

Exhibit 7–2 Evaluation Criteria

Pharmacy Risk: Evaluation Criteria for Medical Group or Health System

1. What is the group's experience with other forms of capitation and shared risk arrangements? How successful have they been with these agreements?
2. What has been the group's pharmacy experience over the last two years? How have the drug costs been trending?
3. Does the contract allow for adjustments in funding due to inflation or new drug technology?
4. How are injectable drug costs managed and by whom?
5. Who is/are the patient population(s) included in the pharmacy risk arrangements? Are they large enough to spread the risk?
6. Has the patient population been clearly defined? For example, does the contract include only HMO patients or is it for an entire commercial population?
7. Is there a clinical pharmacist on staff or can the group contract with a consultant pharmacist in the management of these risk arrangements?
8. Will the health plan provide electronic prescription claims data? Does the group have the necessary information technology infrastructure to manage their drug claims data?
9. What are the current pharmacy benefit designs in which the patients are enrolled? For example, how many patients are under closed formularies, tiered copayments, or have annual caps on the drug benefit? Does the contract allow for adjustments in funding due to significant changes in benefit design?

---

tings," in *Principles of Pharmacoeconomics*.[5]) Today, however, it is still safe to say that pharmacoeconomic analyses have had less impact on pharmacy benefits and formulary decisions than many would have hoped. Reasons for a slower-than-expected rate of pharmacy adoption of pharmacoeconomics include the following:

- the low scientific quality of especially early attempts leading to a distrust of discipline (as simply "cost justification")
- the ethical dilemma of the predominate sponsor of the research being pharmaceutical manufacturers

- the highly statistical methodologies that are difficult to understand and emulate
- the evolving methodologies and unresolved methodological issues (e.g., the weight given to quality-of-life in pharmacoeconomic assessments of medical technologies)
- the remaining questions regarding valuing lost productivity, human life, and other concepts that are difficult to put into monetary terms
- the demonstrations that cost savings are often realized outside of pharmacy benefit

Nonetheless, health plans are paying increasing attention to pharmacoeconomics. Formulary committees now typically include health economists who understand pharmacoeconomic methodologies—e.g., cost-minimization, cost-effectiveness, cost-utility, and cost-benefit analyses— and who can competently judge the scientific validity of the studies. These new formulary members help pharmacy benefit managers understand relative "economic value" of new therapies. Pharmacoeconomic models are beginning to be used to project the economic impact of adding new agents as well as to predict economic value. Finally, on the basis of these analyses, organizations are beginning to look for plan savings across budgets. These trends are likely to continue.

PHARMACOECONOMIC CASE STUDY

The following case involving the prophylactic use of acyclovir to prevent herpes in immunocompromised HIV patients reflects this approach.

Background

Managing pharmacy risk should involve understanding when and how to use pharmaceuticals in a cost-effective manner. Much has been written in recent years about the emerging discipline of pharmacoeconomics, a specific subbranch of health economics that attempts to determine the economic value of alternative pharmaceutical therapies. When properly applied, pharmaco-economics can be an important tool for medical groups/

health systems that are contemplating or are already involved with pharmacy risk arrangements. Rigorous quantitative analyses may sometimes lead the group at risk to take steps or to formulate clinical guidelines that are initially counterintuitive or not readily identifiable absent the analyses.

An illustrative example of the role of this type of analysis comes from the Department of Pharmaceutical Services, University Hospital, University of Nebraska. During the fall of 1994, Lori Murante, Pharm.D., Head of Clinical Pharmacy Services, and Dean Collier, Pharm.D., Assistant Professor, College of Pharmacy, were interested in the cost impact of using acyclovir prophylactically for herpes simplex virus (HSV) in immunocompromised patients such as those often seen in the University of Nebraska transplant center. Drs. Murante and Collier developed a pharmacoeconomic model to compare the economic value of prophylactically treating patients at risk for HSV relative to treating episodically (i.e., only when they had an outbreak).

The Model

The model was developed from a medical decision tree taken from published clinical studies of prophylactic and episodic use of acyclovir for HSV. These clinical studies indicated differences in the probability of major and minor episodes from these two treatment alternatives (see Table 7–1).

These major and minor episodes of HSV were identified in the University of Nebraska Hospital records, and then the medical resources associated with each episode were identified and costed using University of Nebraska costs. These costs are presented in Tables 7–2 and 7–3 below.

Table 7–1 Outcome Probabilities of Prophylaxis vs. Episodic Treatment of HSV

Outcome	Prophylaxis	Episodic
Major Episode	0.015	0.035
Minor Episode	0.09	0.32
No Episode	0.895	0.645

Table 7-2 Costs for Minor HSV Episode, Uncomplicated Treatment

Resource	Prob.	Unit Cost	Units	Cost
Hospital (general ward)	1	$361.00	3	$1,083.00
IV Acyclovir (1,050mg)	1	84.71	3	254.13
Daily Labs	1	66.81	3	200.43
Culture Tzanck	1	33.21	1	33.21
Minor Episode Total				$1,570.77

The estimated cost for each treatment alternative is found by multiplying the outcome probabilities of each event (major episode, minor episode, and no episode) times the total cost of the resources consumed during each episode, plus the therapy costs associated with each treatment alternative, and then summing. The summed totals are then compared to determine the estimated difference in total costs between each therapeutic alternative.

Results

The model projected total per patient costs for episodic acyclovir treatment in immunocompromised patients is $811.76. The total projected costs for prophylaxis treatment computed to $550.79. The estimated difference is $260.97 per patient, where a positive number represents a savings for prophylaxis over episodic treatment. Over 100 patients, then, this difference could account for over $26,000. A number of sensitivity analyses were performed on the model and determined that the model

Table 7-3 Costs for Major HSV Episode, Complicated Treatment

Resource	Prob.	Unit Cost	Units	Cost
Hospital (liver surgery care unit)	1	$961.00	7	$6,727.00
IV Acyclovir (2,100 mg)	1	169.42	7	1,185.94
Daily Labs	1	66.81	7	467.67
Liver Biopsy	0.6	363.48	1	218.09
Endoscopy	0.4	386.73	1	154.69
Culture, HSV, CMV, Fungal	1	78.46	1	78.46
Major Episode Total				$8,831.85

results were robust across a range of model manipulations. Key sensitivities were the probability of a major episode and the cost of a major episode. Interestingly, the model was insensitive to the cost of oral acyclovir.

On the basis of this analysis, Drs. Murante and Collier determined that prophylactic acyclovir treatment would be cost effective in their hospital. This information was then used to develop appropriate use protocols for their hospital that call for prophylactic treatment of immunocompromised patients. These protocols are revisited each year to ensure that the findings remain current, both relative to the most recent literature and consistent with hospital records' analyses.

REMAINING ISSUES

There are a number of remaining issues regarding the adoption and integration of pharmacoeconomic thinking and analyses into pharmacy management. These include the following:

- the extent to which pharmacy benefit decisions will be governed by strict considerations of cost effectiveness (e.g., as in the Oregon Medicaid experiment)
- the degree to which our society will accept the rigorous challenge of basing health decisions on cost-effectiveness criteria
- the ability of, and incentives for, pharmacy administrators to look beyond the pharmacy budget to the entire medical budget and "offsets"
- the continued growth in size and legitimacy of a pharmacoeconomic discipline
- the fuller integration of health economists into health plan decision making
- the appearance of alternatives to pharmaceutical industry-sponsored studies

As these issues are resolved, we should expect pharmacy risk management to increase the utilization of pharmacoeconomics.

REFERENCES

1. K.E. Warner and B.R. Luce. 1982. *Cost-Benefit and Cost-Effectiveness Analysis in Health Care* (Ann Arbor, MI: Health Administration Press).
2. J.L. Bootman et al. 1996. *Principles of Pharmacoeconomics* Cincinnati OH: Harvey Whitney Books Company.
3. B. Spilker. 1996. *Quality of Life and Pharmacoeconomics in Clinical Trials*, 2d ed. Philadelphia: Lippincott-Raven Publishers).
4. A. Wimo et al. 1998. *Health Economics of Dementia* (Chichester, U.K.: John Wiley & Sons).
5. A. Stergachis et al. 1996. The application of pharmacoeconomics in managed healthcare settings, In *Principles of Pharma-coeconomics*, eds. J.L. Bootman et al.,242–256. Cincinnati OH: Harvey Whitney Books Company.

SUGGESTED READINGS

Facts and Figures. 1998. *Novartis Pharmacy Benefit Report.*

Hoescht Marion Roussel, HMO-PPO/Medicare/Medicaid Digest. 1998. *Managed Care Digest Series.*

"IMS Health Reports Managed Care Programs Control Nearly Two-thirds of the U.S. Retail Prescription Drug Market," (Press Release).

Merck Medco Managed Care, LLC. 1999. *Managing Pharmacy Benefit Costs.*

"Trends and Forecasts," *Novartis Pharmacy Benefit Report*, 1998.

1999. Data show golden age for the pharmaceutical industry. *Drug Benefit Trends*, April, 13–17.

CHAPTER 8

Answers to Practical Legal Questions

David C. Main, Esq., and T. Lane Macalester, Esq.

What Should Be the Advice to Providers Getting Involved in Capitation? Where Should They Be Focused?

Perhaps surprisingly, concerns about capitation have less to do with the legal aspects of this type of payment arrangement and more to do with prudent business practices. Too many providers engage in capitation ill prepared, lacking fundamental financial and administrative information that destines capitation to failure. More specifically, providers should be asking themselves the following questions:

- Do you know precisely what you are at risk for? What is the scope of services? What is "carved out" of the capitation to reduce inappropriate risk?
- How was the capitation calculated? What are the underlying assumptions used? Where did they come from? Are they based on actual experience or were they imported from another geographic region under optimal conditions?
- How long do you want to be involved in the capitated arrangement? What is your tolerance for the risk? Can you withstand the ups and downs for two years, three years, or more? How important is the overall relationship with the payer?

Providers really need to understand the payer perspective. That translates into getting a good actuary involved, understanding precisely how

121

products will be marketed, and getting legal help from attorneys who understand both the payer and provider side of the equation.

What Do Providers Worry about Too Much, from a Legal Perspective?

Lawyers are paid to worry about a lot of things on the legal side, on behalf of clients—various health care providers. Providers tend to become consumed with certain legal nuances to protect their risk rather than spending the time prior to contract negotiations to define services, understand the financial terms, and negotiate better arrangements. Those aspects pay off far more than some extra "legal language." However, there are still a number of other things to worry about. These concerns include:

- Is the term of the contract appropriate? It needs to be long enough, such as two to three years, for providers to gain the right experience, but not so long or restrictive that the provider is locked in under an adverse contract. A contract can be longer term if "mini-outs" are structured into the arrangement. For example, some clients have negotiated periodic reviews and focused renegotiation to ensure that the contract stays on track for both sides.
- Is there exclusivity or channeling involved? What is the size of the network? What are the reasonable expectations for growth? These, again, are not strictly legal issues, but clients should be counseled to understand fully how the delivery system is structured (or not) around the capitation agreement. If the delivery system, through exclusivity or some other form of channeling, does not support the build up in volume, the provider is going to struggle with the capitation.
- Do the physicians understand the protocols and clinical direction of the contractual arrangement? Are they committed to following them? Are there controls to enforce that behavior? It is hard to break down the clinical requirements of various contracts that may differ from one another. Nonetheless, there is not enough attention paid by clinicians to this important area. Physicians are creating potential legal liability with the health plan member and the payer when they fail to follow protocols, referral procedures, appeal rights, etc. Many providers tend to generalize in this area, and struggle through, disregarding some important dimensions of the care management process.

Capitation Is Complex, with Many Nuances. Moreover, Payer-Provider Relationships Have Become Less Predictable. It is Difficult To Anticipate Every Contingency. How Do You See Providers Handling This "Reality," Both in Negotiations and Contract Writing? Do You Define As Much As Possible on the Front End?

If the right preparation is done on the front end relating to analysis, research, and reviewing data, most, if not all, of the critical issues can be addressed explicitly in the contract. Mature, well-represented providers entering into capitation have negotiated solid, sophisticated arrangements that will serve them well. Even these providers, though, often find that they cannot anticipate everything. There are always unknown factors that are either not divulged by the health plan or are not anticipated by either party. For example, the application of out-of-network utilization to incentive funds, or credits and rebates for prescription drugs to a shared risk pool are merely two areas that often get overlooked. As another example, reinsurance has many dimensions that can be interpreted differently in the reconciliation process. In a good provider-payer relationship, compromises on interpretation often will be worked out in the interests of both parties and the spirit of the arrangement.

In today's competitive, cost-driven health care arena, though, short-term results are typically critical. Relationships are developed in the context of one to two-year timeframes. Hence, there is increasing gamesmanship and manipulation occurring around these contractual nuances to garner stronger financial results. We are advising that providers be very cautious about entering into longer-term arrangements and attempt to incorporate viable exit provisions in the event that the arrangement becomes completely unworkable or financially ruinous to either party.

How Do Regulators View Capitation? What Concerns Should Providers Have Related to Legal Compliance with State and Federal Statutes?

The regulatory environment varies from state to state. A number of states have addressed capitation expressly and effectively regulate the assumption of risk by providers through statute, rules, interpretations, and opinions. Frankly, some regulation of capitation is clearly supported in the legal system, while other aspects of oversight are supported by regulators' general sphere of power and influence. Consequently, a provider operating in that context needs to be aware that capitation will be scrutinized. On the other hand, there are a larger number of states that have not addressed the issue. Capitation is either not prevalent or has not been an issue of concern to regulators there. Insurance is regulated at the state level through departments of insurance and other regulatory bodies. The federal government does not directly enter this arena other than through the impact of the Employee Retirement Income Security Act (ERISA) and its oversight of the immense Medicare and Medicaid programs. To the degree there is a conflict with state regulations on the topic, federal law may preempt state law.

While virtually every state addresses the concept of capitation in the context of managed care arrangements with providers, there is not uniformity among jurisdictions as to the level of risk that may be transferred to providers or, at least, acceptable without prior regulatory review of the agreement. Regardless of statutory requirements on the topic, enforcement and interpretation of such statutes by state authorities may shift over time, particularly if a jurisdiction experienced insolvency by a significant provider group that caused public concern about continuity of providing health care to consumers.

Regulatory agencies that address the concept of risk bearing among providers generally adhere to the policy that the managed care organization is the entity directly regulated, not the provider. In other words, if there are particular terms that the statute requires be part of the provider agreement with the managed care organization, regulators will hold the managed care organization liable for any noncompliance. Typically, these statutory requirements are of a financial (net worth) or even programmatic nature, such as quality assurance standards. In a minority of states, there is the potential that a risk bearing provider may be required to obtain an insurance license, irrespective of the insurance or HMO licensed entity with which it contracts.

How Do Various Regulatory Requirements Directly Impact the Capitation Arrangement with a Provider and How the Provider Operates under It?

Aside from the overall context referenced previously, providers have to face certain genuine and practical requirements. They include:

- Financial security. Providers will need to provide deposits, letters of credit, or other secured assets in some cases to support their assumption of risk.

- Administrative capabilities. Payers are being held accountable for ensuring that the provider is prepared and capable of handling risk assumption, administratively. That means being well organized in terms of business functions, use of technology, information flow, etc. The personnel are well intended, but there is still far too much short-term functioning that occurs on a day-to-day basis. While there has been growth in the sophistication of capitated arrangements, there has not been the same parallel development in provider administrative capabilities.
- Contractual requirements. Certain provisions related to terms such as health plan member protection and continuity of care must be included in the contract between the payer and provider, regardless of how the provider feels about it.

In general, provider offices should be prepared to understand the myriad of operational considerations in providing health care services to patients enrolled in managed care plans. These considerations span financial, administrative, and contractual aspects of a provider's business, including:

- Verification of patient (member) enrollment in a health plan;
- Collection of appropriate copayment from the member;
- Adherence to prior authorization and/or referral protocols;
- Compilation of any encounter data reporting requirements; and
- Accommodation of any member service requirements (such as 24-hour coverage and prompt scheduling of appointments).

Managed care plans typically vary from each other in these types of requirements, which complicates implementation. Consequently, providers must have the capacity to administer specific protocols on a payer-by-payer basis.

What Is the Impact of a Provider Accepting Capitation and Then Subcapitating Other Providers? Is That Subsequent Capitation Regulated?

The short answer to this question is that subcapitation is regulated as well. Regulators and payers are both concerned about "weak links" in the system. Even though one or more providers are capable of assuming risk, a weak provider can undermine the rest of the system and directly impact care being delivered to members. Therefore, accountability goes down the line. The requirements that were referenced previously, perhaps modified to some degree depending upon the nature of the subcapitation, will be applicable to these other providers.

Health Plans and Insurers Have Different Levels of Competence in Their Administrative Systems Supporting Capitation and Related Risk Arrangements. How Can a Provider Address Payer "Incompetence" or Malfeasance in This Critical Area?

This is probably one of the toughest, most challenging issues with which to contend. In the early years of the managed care industry, payers, for a variety of reasons, limited their product offerings and concentrated on a limited number of payment arrangements. Their administrative systems were rudimentary, but their operating requirements were as well. More-over, some companies clearly chose to focus on capitation of one type or another and built their administrative and other capabilities around it. In effect, they made capitation a "core competency." As problems developed with capitation, payers addressed the issues with providers directly, per-sonally, and with some urgency.

Today's environment is almost entirely different. It is much more complex. Greater numbers and types of products are offered. Payment arrangements are much more heterogeneous in comparison to 10 or 15 years ago. Payers have grown rapidly, creating strains on their administrative capabilities generally. On top of that, there have been a number of mergers and acquisitions, creating a patchwork of administrative systems operating within the same corporate environment. The result is trouble for many capitated providers. It is a fair statement that health plans probably intend to administer the capitated arrangements properly, but they have too little time, people, and financial resources devoted to the task to deliver consistently. The result is "incompetence" or malfeasance, regardless of the intent.

In this environment, with those realities, providers must assume that payer performance will be less than desired and required. Providers need to build in protections up front to avoid harmful battles down the road when payer "incompetence" directly affects the financial performance of the capitated arrangement. The protections include the following, at a mini-mum:

- An audit of the payers relevant, supporting administrative systems. This may best be done by an outside, expert organization with proven audit and review capabilities in this area.
- Establishment of performance standards related to the contract related to data, information, reconciliations, reviews, contracting, etc. These standards may start at one level and change over time to correlate with payer readiness. The initial level of performance, though, must satisfy threshold provider needs.
- Requirement of valid, meaningful, quarterly data reporting. This reporting, though, should be more than a raw data dump. The information should be formatted to be readable and reviewed by the appropriate group for content. The reports should encompass enrollment, member "adds and deletes," capitation payments made, fund balances, benefit changes, marketing plans, etc. The qualitative information is just as important as the fundamental numbers.

What Financial and Service Exposures Are Created for Providers and Practitioners Involved in Capitation, Emanating from the Very Visible Organizational and Financial Struggles of Large PPMCs Such As FPA and Medpartners?

First, it is important to note that the regulatory authorities in the states in which these companies operate may hold the health plans or insurers that make capitation payments to these groups responsible for ensuring that the groups have the financial solvency and contractual obligations to deliver the services for which they are being capitated. As a result, in situations where the groups have run out of money, some major health plans have had to make additional payments directly to providers (i.e., in addition to the capitation payments already paid to the groups) to ensure that they were paid for their services and continued to deliver them. While they may not have had a contractual obligation to do so, regulators may exert pressure on the health plans to rectify what amounts to an insolvency situation and ensure that health plan members are not left without service or the burden of paying for the services themselves. Thus, individual practitioners and members have been protected, to some degree, even in the midst of financial chaos, in order to protect ultimately the members enrolled with those provider groups.

As a result, and especially in those states imposing these requirements, both the regulators and the health plans that capitate major provider groups will increase their scrutiny of providers—their financial health and their administrative capabilities. In general, regulators have been establishing requirements for capitating health plans in these areas for years due to previous problems of this sort. The magnitude of these recent episodes probably has injected more caution into the health plans that found themselves financially responsible in order to create stability for their members. They will, of course, be more guarded about entering into new arrangements of this kind.

Finally, financial problems in the payment of physicians under such capitation arrangements create issues for the individual practitioner or practice, relating to their continuing obligation to provide care when not receiving compensation for their services. Physicians should carefully attend to the language of their agreements describing their obligations to continue medical treatment under these circumstances.

Does Capitation Increase a Provider's Exposure to Professional Malpractice?

Exposure to legal liability actually stems from a variety of sources for a provider, such as: poor clinical judgment, inadequate fact-finding, poor communication, or inappropriate expectations, as well as from the perverse response to incentives by withholding, delaying, or minimizing care. Clearly, in today's charged environment related to "what managed care does or does not do," more people have a heightened awareness of how capitation or other related economic incentives could diminish the quality of care, therefore creating increased legal exposure for the provider. Some providers, unfortunately, do respond all too well to the incentives put before them, whether that encourages them to increase unnecessary care or reduce the amount of care necessary.

On the other hand, providers have a number of factors to influence them to provide the appropriate care, even when capitated. Their own pledge and personal integrity, their personal interest in the welfare of the patient, the real exposure to malpractice, and finally, the quality management system of the capitating payer all create an environment that is conducive to good care. Payers have a responsibility to create strong quality management systems that seek out and identify incidences and patterns of underutilization.

Providers, in fact, should scrutinize how well developed those systems are before accepting capitation. If they are inadequately developed, providers should defer or forgo the capitated arrangement.

In a logical, rational environment, capitation should not, in and of itself, create increased professional exposure, particularly when the arrangement has been well negotiated and structured. Of course, the world around us does not always behave rationally. People perceive things to be a certain way—that capitated providers are over mindful of cash registers as they diagnose and prescribe treatments. To the degree that a plaintiff's attorney can create that picture and reinforce it, then there is going to be some exposure that emanates from capitation. That's a reality. People need to focus on doing the right thing, creating the right context so that good, appropriate care focused on the patient is provided. With capitation, that may well mean that more appropriate, effective treatments and approaches are utilized because fixed income arrangements tend to encourage efficiencies rather than the opposite, singular incentive in a fee-for-service model for reward merely by rendering a greater volume of services.

Do Various "Managed Care Safeguards" Such As a Bill of Rights or External Panel Reviews Impact Provider Liability Issues, Particularly Related to Capitation?

This question requires a dual response. In a "rational" world, these additional safeguards will not do that much to diminish liability for providers. Risk of liability is diminished if providers remain current in their practice, managing expectations, communicating well, and following up quickly and appropriately. Those are the best safeguards for providers, either inside or outside capitated arrangements. Because this is not always a rational environment, many people in this country are concerned with the potential for adverse care due to economics driving decisions. Consequently, we are not going to conquer some of this mania until we establish some additional safeguards and assurances for a public that is increasingly covered by some type of managed care arrangement. The health plan trade associations, a number of employers, and others may not agree, but we need to address people's anxieties. Many health plans, particularly the best run ones with a strong history of quality, are already doing much in this arena, so these public efforts serve as comforting, albeit redundant, measures.

The Health Care Reimbursement and Payment Arena Is Closely Regulated by Laws Related to Self-Referral, False Claims, Fraud and Abuse, and Whistle-Blowing among Others. Do These Apply in the Capitated World As Well? What Are the Most Relevant Provisions Here?

From an attorney's perspective, this is one of the more intriguing questions. The health care world is under intense scrutiny from many angles—the Health Care Financing Administration (HCFA), the Office of Inspector General, and the FBI, among others. Notably, much of the scrutiny focuses on "excesses" stemming from the perverse incentives of fee-for-service or cost reimbursement. There is fertile ground that is keeping federal, state, and local authorities busy just in the traditional reimbursement arena. For example, the Columbia investigations cover a wide range of compliance issues and involve hundreds of officials and staff. Clearly, providers now understand the concern and have internally tightened their procedures, established formal compliance programs, and adopted a more proactive stance generally.

Capitation, by its nature, does not invoke a traditional billing and claims payment process, as we know it. However, many laws were originally based on conventional concepts. At the same time, we should be prepared to see the application of some of these laws to capitation and the development of others, assuming that capitation does expand as a payment mode. The best protection against this expansion of legal authority is entering into risk arrangements that are prudent for the provider as businessperson. This requires the provider to become educated about the office's administrative capacity required to implement the arrangement. It also means assessing the financial responsibility required for the patient population served, including protecting against catastrophic medical expenses and, in the case of subcontracted providers, understanding the ramifications if an "upstream" provider fails financially. With this knowledge, the provider is prepared to evaluate the quality of how the capitation is structured, the payers and providers involved, the controls in place, and a consistent respect for the intent and spirit of the law.

SUGGESTED READING

Could capitation's legal 'gray areas' put you at risk? 1998. *Capitation Management Report* 5, No. 7: 97–101.

CHAPTER 9

How Deep Is Your Risk Pool?

Jon A. Brunsberg, MBA

INTERNAL REIMBURSEMENT MECHANISMS

Whether a health plan is capitating a physician group or an integrated delivery system, there may be a significant number of individual physicians and multiple entities participating under a full capitation arrangement. When entering into such an agreement, there should be proactive planning regarding the structure of reimbursement for services provided by these individual providers and how deviations from expected budgets will be handled. Handling deviations is typically called surplus and deficit allocation.

Basic Principles

In developing an internal reimbursement mechanism, the following are the basic principles that should be addressed:

- The reimbursement mechanism should provide for an equitable distribution of the capitation dollars. This is a challenge since each party tries to maximize its income within the constraint that the total capitation income is the upper bound for payments to individual providers.
- The reimbursement mechanism should provide incentives to control overall utilization and reward efficiency and quality in the provision of medical care. Likewise, the mechanism should not excessively harm individual providers because of circumstances beyond their control.
- Adequate provision should be made for services that the network will not provide. For example, the mechanism should address the costs for

131

out-of-area emergency care if these services are included in the capitation.

- A risk absorption approach should be established to protect cash flow in the event that costs, on a predefined provider payment system, exceed the capitation.
- The mechanism should not be so overly complex as to confuse participating providers or create an excessive administrative burden. There is often intense pressure to create the perfect risk-sharing model, only to find that the provider group is not able to administer the model.

General Structure

The general structure of a reimbursement mechanism can be thought of as having two elements:

1. Provider Payment—The provider payment approach defines how providers will be paid on a day-to-day basis.
2. Risk Sharing—The risk-sharing approach determines how providers are ultimately paid for services and defines the process of how surplus dollars are distributed (the settlement process).

The relative importance of these two components depends upon the structure of the provider entity contracting with the health plan. The combination of the two elements must be able to absorb risk if resource consumption is greater than expected.

At a minimum, this may require a withhold (explicit risk sharing) or an aggressive fee schedule relative to the capitation level (implicit risk sharing). In either case, there should be expectations that the capitation is sufficient to cover the day-to-day payments to providers. Any surplus or withhold dollars can be distributed within the risk-sharing mechanism. Alternatively, if all services covered within a global capitation are subcapitated to various providers, the risk-sharing component may be a mute point.

External Pool Allocations

In developing a budget for the apportionment of the capitation, there will likely be several categories of expenses that fall outside of the capabilities of the participating providers. Allocations for these external expenses should be established prospectively to avoid misunderstandings. The following are several items that should be considered in developing a budget:

- Contribution to Surplus—In particular, a provider entity may set aside monies to fund a surplus reserve. These monies can be used to retire start-up expenses, fund capital expenses such as computer software, or address statutory reserve (net worth) requirements.
- Administrative Expense Allocation—For a provider organization, administrative costs will need to be funded.
- Excess Loss Coverage—If the health plan does not provide coverage within the capitation contract, the provider group may purchase or self-fund excess loss coverage. The premium to purchase this coverage (or allocation for self-funding) needs to be allocated from the capitation. Reinsurance recoveries would be allocated in a similar manner.
- Non-Network Medical Service Expenses—There will likely be a portion of the medical services performed by nonparticipating providers. These would include emergency care, referrals to nonparticipating subspecialists, and in the case of point-of-service products, the costs of member self-referrals to non-network physicians.

Depending on the product, a portion of the capitation revenue should be set aside to cover these anticipated expenses. Unused funds would be available for distribution, and deficiencies in this allocation need to be funded during the settlement process.

- Subcapitation Payments—The provider group may transfer responsibility for certain services to a third party in return for a per member capitation. Services that are often capitated include mental health and substance abuse services and reference lab services. Specialty physician and disease management capitations are becoming more common, as well.
- Shared Risk Pool Exposure—The capitation agreement with the plan may include a shared risk incentive arrangement for hospital, pharmacy, and/or ancillary services. To the extent that the provider group may be liable for deficits in this fund, provision should be made to

accommodate these potential losses. This exposure can be handled as an external pool allocation or within the settlement process of the risk-sharing mechanism.

Once external pool allocations have been defined, the remainder of the capitation is available for services provided by participating providers.

Risk-Sharing Options

Risk sharing is fundamental to developing an internal reimbursement mechanism under capitation. The risk-sharing approach should be developed to encourage the alignment of the incentives of participating providers. Consistent with the basic principles outlined above, the risk-sharing approach should:

- provide cash flow protection to the capitated provider group, and
- promote the cost-effective delivery of quality health care.

A simple example of a risk-sharing approach, for an IPA network, would be to implement a withhold. Ideally, the withhold would be set at such a level that the likelihood of a cash deficit is fairly small.

For example, if the physician capitation is $40, and the withhold is 15 percent, then expected payments throughout the year would be $34 pmpm. Any gains could be distributed on the basis of payments withheld throughout the year.

Table 9–1 illustrates potential results under this arrangement.

As a risk-sharing approach, this model has the advantage of being administratively simple, and in aggregate, provides some incentives to control utilization. The biggest disadvantage is that the incentives for an individual provider to control utilization are diluted because utilization and ultimate reimbursement are still highly correlated on an individual basis. Also, specific problem areas are not highlighted by the use of this model.

The following section describes two basic risk-sharing approaches in the context of a global capitation internal reimbursement mechanism. Presented are examples of a one-pool settlement (Table 9–2) and a two-pool settlement (Table 9–3) when actual claim experience varies both positively and negatively from expected levels.

Table 9–1 Distribution Scenarios (PMPM)

	Scenario 1	Scenario 2	Scenario 3
Expected	$40.00	$40.00	$40.00
Actual[1]	38.00	40.00	42.00
Gain/(Loss)	2.00	0.00	(2.00)
Withholds[2]	5.70	6.00	6.30
Distribution[3]	7.70	6.00	4.30

[1]Assuming reimbursement at target schedule (before withhold
  reduction).
[2]15% of actual PMPM. For simplicity, assumes all providers subject
to withhold. In reality, some providers (e.g., non-network referrals)
would not be subject to withholds.
[3]Sum of the withholds and the gain/(loss).

For simplicity all services are assumed to occur in-network and are subject to withholds. The tables walk-through scenarios where actual medical expenses are at, above, or below the budgeted level, given a predefined per service reimbursement. Results are measured in relation to the predefined reimbursement.

IN SUMMARY

To ensure reasonable long-term reimbursement levels in a capitated environment, an organization accepting risk should first ensure that, in aggregate, its capitated agreements provide for reasonable fee-for-service equivalent reimbursement rates. Internal reimbursement for the services of individual providers should be structured to provide some cash flow protection to the provider as well as to promote the cost-effective delivery of medical care. Although there are a number of variations to consider in developing a provider reimbursement and risk-sharing mechanism, this chapter has presented an example that may be used as a starting point for discussions within a particular provider organization.

As with most facets of managed care, a reimbursement mechanism cannot be developed in a vacuum. Care should be taken to coordinate these efforts with the provider group's utilization management, quality assurance, and information systems functions.

Table 9–2 Year-End Reconciliation Illustration—One-Pool Approach

	Claims at Expected Levels	Claims Above Expected Levels	Claims Below Expected Levels
Gain/(Loss) Calculation	($100.00)	($110.00)	($90.00)
• Medical Expense Pool Budget	$100.00	$100.00	$100.00
– Hospital Expenses (net of 15% withhold)	$46.75	51.00	42.50
– Physician Expenses (net of 15% withhold)	36.55	40.80	32.30
– Net Reinsurance Costs	2.00	2.00	2.00
• Gain/(Loss)	$14.70	$6.20	$23.20
Withhold Distribution			
• Total Withheld			
– Hospital Partner	$8.25	$9.00	$7.50
– Physician Group	6.45	7.20	5.70
• Withhold Distributed			
– Hospital Partner	$8.25	$3.44	$7.50
– Physician Group	6.45	2.76	5.70
• Percent of Withhold Distributed	100%	38.3%	100%
Excess Gain Distribution			
• Excess Gain	$0.00	$0.00	$10.00
• Hospital Partner (40%)	0.00	0.00	4.00
• Physician Group (40%)	0.00	0.00	4.00
• Reserve (20%)	0.00	0.00	2.00

Total Distribution			
• Hospital Partner	$8.25	$3.44	$11.50
• Physician Group	6.45	2.76	9.70
• Reserve	0.00	0.00	2.00
Percent of Desired Reimbursement			
• Hospital Partner	100%	90.7%	108.0%
• Physician Group	100%	90.7%	110.5%

Table 9–3 Year-End Reconciliation Illustration—Two-Pool Approach

	Claims at Expected Levels ($100.00)	Claims Slightly Above Expected Levels ($110.00)	Claims Signif. Above Exp. Levels ($125.00)	Claims Below Exp. Levels ($90.00)
Gain/(Loss) Calculation				
• Hospital Pool Budget	$55.00	$55.00	$55.00	$55.00
— Hospital Expenses	54.00	59.00	69.00	49.00
— Net Reinsurance Costs	1.00	1.00	1.00	1.00
— Gain/(Loss)	0.00	(5.00)	(15.00)	5.00
• Physician Pool Budget	$43.00	$43.00	$43.00	$43.00
— Physician Expenses	42.00	47.00	52.00	37.00
— Net Reinsurance Costs	1.00	1.00	1.00	1.00
— Gain/(Loss)	0.00	(5.00)	(10.00)	5.00
Gain/(Loss) Distribution				
• Hospital Pool	$0.00	($5.00)	(15.00)	$5.00
— Hospital Partner	0.00	(5.00)	(15.00)	2.50
— Physician Group	0.00	0.00	0.00	2.50
• Physician Pool	$0.00	($5.00)	(10.00)	$5.00
— Hospital Partner	0.00	0.00	(2.20)	0.00
— Physician Group	0.00	(5.00)	(7.80)	5.00
Total Distribution				

Hospital Partner	$0.00	($5.00)	(17.20)	$2.50
Physician Group	0.00	(5.00)	(7.80)	7.50
Percent of Desired Reimbursement				
Hospital Partner	100%	91.5%	75.1%	105.1%
Physician Group	100%	89.3%	85.0%	120.3%

CHAPTER 10

Incurred Claim Reserves and Things That Go Bump in the Night

The recent financial problems of several health plans can be attributed to poor estimates of incurred claims and claim reserves. Increasing the balance sheet reserve is the first step in fixing a reserve problem, but organizations in this position will also likely have other, more difficult problems to address due to business decisions already made based on understated estimates of incurred claims. Some of these problems could prove to be fatal. Accurate estimates of the incurred claims used to set claim reserves provide insurers and at-risk provider organizations the basis for long-term strategic planning.

Balance sheet claim reserves often are called IBNR reserves (incurred but not received). This is somewhat of a misnomer in that the reserve amount usually accounts for both the amount not yet received and the amount received, but waiting to be paid. A more accurate term would be IBNP (incurred but not paid).

There are several problem areas to beware of in making incurred claim and claim reserve estimates. It is also important to retroactively assess how accurate these estimates were.

POTENTIAL PROBLEMS

The most common problem is a sporadic pattern of claims payment. As discussed below, the IBNP reserve usually is developed from a lag analysis. Such an analysis can only provide reasonable results when the historical claim payments exhibit a pattern that predicts future claim payments. Therefore, claim backlogs (the level of claims waiting to be paid) must be monitored and adjustments made to the lag analysis when appropriate.

The impact of claim backlogs also can be eliminated by basing the lag analysis on date of receipt instead of date of payment. One drawback of a received lag analysis is that it is imperative to have all received claims entered into the system by a strictly observed cutoff date, ideally with a system determination of the claim adjudication.

Another common problem is how to treat large claims. Such claims can "trick" a lag analysis into thinking that claims are being paid faster or slower than they really are. In such cases, performing the analysis without these claims will better predict future claims. It is important to remember to add the large claim back in when stating total incurred claims.

Predicting IBNP reserves is also difficult when a product has not been offered for long or has a small membership base. In these cases, incurred claims are sometimes estimated by using the lag completion factors for other blocks of business or by applying an expected loss ratio. It is important to monitor estimates made in this way for reasonability and to switch to a lag analysis as soon as possible.

LAG ANALYSIS

The most common method used to calculate the IBNP is to review the historical claim payment patterns for each date of service (i.e., the lag between the service date and the paid date) and project the amounts remaining to be paid. There are many variations of this method, but they are all commonly referred to as lag analyses. A lag analysis consists of six key steps. These steps and a simplified example are described below. (The analysis usually would be made separately for each line of business and often also by different categories of service.)

- **Step 1.** Gather the historical claim payments by date of service and date paid. Because of the shape of the resulting report, these reports are often called claim triangles. The example presented here has been simplified by assuming that all claims are completely paid by the end of the third month following the incurred date. Once the claim triangle data is gathered, the cumulative claims paid are calculated for each date of service.

# Months After Incurral	Paid Claims By Incurral Month				Cumulative Paid Claims By Incurral Month			
	Sept.	Oct.	Nov.	Dec.	Sept.	Oct.	Nov.	Dec.
0	$200	$240	$200	$350	$200	$240	$200	$350
1	450	540	600		650	780	800	
2	100	120			750	900		
3	50				800			

- **Step 2.** Calculate the percentage change in cumulative paid claims each month, called the completion ratio. Many different formulas are used to calculate these ratios. In this example, the arithmetic average of all dates of service in the analysis has been assumed. The completion factor for each service date is then calculated as the product of each of the monthly completion ratios. The completion factor is an estimate of the percentage of total incurred claims that already have been paid, or how "complete" paid claims are. In the example, it is estimated that claims paid within one month following the incurred date are 82 percent of what the amount will ultimately be when claims have been completely paid.

# Months After Incurral	Completion Ratios				Average Completion Ratios	Completion Factors
	Sept.	Oct.	Nov.	Dec.		
0	.31	.31	.25	--	$.29^2$	.24
1	$.87^1$	.87			.87	$.82^4$
2	.94				.94	.94
3	--				--	1.00^3

[1] Based on cumulative paid claims data: .87 = $650 ÷ $750.
[2] Based on completion ratio data: .29 = (.31 + .31 + .25) ÷ 3.
[3] Based on the assumption that 100 percent of claims are paid by the third month following incurral.
[4] .82 = .94 x .87 = (previous month completion factor) x (current month average completion ratio).

- **Step 3.** Calculate the estimated total incurred claims. Since the completion factor indicates how complete the paid claims currently are, total incurred claims equal the cumulative paid claims divided by the completion factor. Incurred claims often are expressed as an amount per covered member in order to see patterns more easily.

Incurral Month	Cumulative Paid Claims Through Dec.[1]	Completion Factor[2]	Initial Incurred Claim Estimate[3]	Members	Cost Per Member
Dec.	$350	.24	$1,458	48	$30
Nov.	800	.82	976	48	20
Oct.	900	.94	957	48	20
Sept.	800	1.00	800	40	20
	$2,850		$4,191		

[1]See Step 1.
[2]See Step 2.
[3]Cumulative paid claims ÷ completion factor.

- **Step 4.** Review the results for potential overrides. Lag analyses are a tool and should not be accepted without critical assessment of the results. This is especially true for the more recent incurral months where the ratios are small and can easily skew the results. In the example, the December estimate of incurred claims is revised assuming the incurred cost per member per month is consistent with prior months. Another common test for overriding inpatient costs is to analyze the historical cost per authorized day.

Incurral Month	Calculated PMPM	PMPM Override	Members	Revised Incurred Claim Estimate[1]
Dec	$30	$20	48	$960
Nov.	20	n/a	48	976
Oct.	20	n/a	48	957
Sept.	20	n/a	40	800
				$3,693

[1]Members x PMPM override or initial estimate if no override.

- **Step 5.** Calculate IBNP liability. The liability for claims not yet paid is equal to the estimate of incurred claims less the amounts that have already been paid prior to the balance sheet date.

Incurral Month	Incurred Claims[1]	Paid As of 12/31[2]	12/31 Unpaid Claim Liability
Dec.	$960	$350	$860
Nov.	976	800	576
Oct.	957	900	307
Sept.	800	800	100
	$3,693	$2,850	$1,843

[1]See Step 4.
[2]See Step 1.

- **Step 6.** Adjust for margin. The amount calculated in Step 5 is a best estimate of the unpaid claim liability. In some cases, this would be the appropriate amount for a lag analysis of IBNP. In most cases, however, actuarial standards of practice require the reserve to provide a measure of conservatism and to include an amount for the cost of adjudicating these delayed claim payments. In the example, a margin of 10 percent has been added.

Best Estimate of Liability	$1,843
10 Percent Margin	184
IBNP Reserve	$2,027

Many organizations do not give enough attention to assessing the accuracy of prior IBNP estimates. The only sure thing is that the estimate is not exactly the right amount. However, it is important to know how wrong it is or whether there is a consistent understatement or overstatement over time.

IBNP estimates for previous balance sheet dates should be restated based on the amount paid between the balance sheet date and the restatement date, plus an estimate for any amount remaining to be paid based on a lag analysis. The restated amount should be compared to the original estimate before and after the margin adjustment. After a few months, restated reserve estimates for medical insurance should remain fairly stable, and reserves more than one year old often do not need to be restated.

This backward look is needed to make timely corrections to the balance sheet, to improve the approach used to make future estimates, and to ensure business decisions are based on a true picture of incurred claim levels.

CHAPTER 11

Conclusion: Physician Leadership Can Turn Pain into Gain

I. David Kibbe, MBA, and Clifford R. Frank, MHSA

In much of health care today, there is a strong tendency to generalize about what works and what does not work. Amid the complexities and confusion in the industry and tremendous pressure to meet financial targets, many professionals are seeking simple, straightforward answers. Is capitation dead or not? Can provider behavior be changed by capitation? Can providers succeed in capitation? Where are the opportunities? Where are the threats? Which payers are the best to work with on capitation? In lieu of satisfactory and clear-cut answers to these and many other capitation-related questions, providers are shying away from it. "Better safe than sorry" comes to mind as a watchword in today's environment related to risk and capitation.

Certainly many providers have been burned by capitation and caution is appropriate. The potential gains of capitation, though, may well be overrun by the anticipated pain of adjusting to capitation, thereby reducing positive change in the health care system. Capitation is, after all, fundamentally about economics shaping human behavior. Those economics can and should be developed and organized in a number of different ways to reflect differences in providers, their capacity for risk, the underlying nature of the population at risk, and the services covered under the risk, among other factors. Historically, for the sake of efficient network development and ease of administration, many payers used a single predominant form of capitation or adaptations of that approach. As the managed care industry has developed and grown more complex, though, the nature and form of capitation has not matured at the same rate and in the same ways. As a consequence, providers have struggled with ill-fitting capitation arrangements, leading to a number of adverse consequences. The pain has been more severe and the gain more limited than anticipated.

The issue is not whether capitation works or not. It has, it does, and it will. Economics focused through capitation arrangements, properly constructed and funded, is a powerful driver for providers to adopt a new mind-set related to managing care. And contrary to many perceptions, that thinking should be, and often is, centered around the patient, the individual member, his or her health, illness prevention, timely intercession, and effective, timely treatment in restoring an individual to health, more so than in a noncapitated environment. The problems have developed where capitation has not been well conceived, providers have not been prepared, contracts have been poorly written, or the underlying risk has not been well evaluated. Often, the economic incentives on individual providers have been too significant. Or the quality management systems to monitor behavior and adverse incidents have not been put in place by payers and providers or used actively by them. Over the past several years particularly, some payers have seen capitation simply as a means of forcing unmanageable risk onto providers at rates, attractive to them but unworkable for the other party. In such cases, capitation is doomed to be troubled and problematic.

Capitation is and will be a powerful and effective driver of positive change in the health care system when both payers and providers consciously work to address challenges that have been identified in the cases and chapters in this book. By doing so, the gain can be achieved and the pain, perhaps not eliminated, but minimized and managed.

THEMES

Active Physician Leadership and Involvement Is Essential

Unfortunately, many physicians recoil with the thought of capitation and stay on the periphery of its development and management. Financial and administrative staff are instrumental in capitation arrangements, but they are not a substitute for the leadership and involvement of physicians. Physician leadership and involvement, too, goes far beyond attending meetings and identifying a medical director. Physician leadership requires that one or several of the physicians develop and maintain a clear vision of the patient care environment and results that they hope to achieve. They reinforce that vision daily and weekly with the meaningful involvement of other physicians and team members. Much more clearly than in other environments operating under more traditional reimbursement, capitation requires physicians who may not choose to lead but are willing, if not eager, to follow the direction set. A group of physicians failing to work together, more or less as a team, will not succeed in a capitated environment in the long term.

Capitation Must Be Viewed as a Fundamental Way of Providing Care and Managing Health, Rather Than Simply as a Financial Payment Mechanism

Clinical behavior, patient education, prevention emphasis, and ambulatory patient care planning all need to be analyzed and redeveloped to provide more effective care under the incentives of capitation. Capitation should spawn a host of clinical discussions and developments—hence, the need for physician leadership and involvement. That involvement extends well beyond board and executive committee meetings to include weekly utilization and quality meetings as well as frequent, ad hoc clinical discussions. In time, capitation leads to a fundamental shift in the way that physicians and other team members view their work, establish priorities, and measure results.

Capitation Must Be Tied to Strong Quality Management Clearly Focused on Potential Problems Emanating from the Capitation Arrangement

Capitation, like any financing, whether fee-for-service or otherwise, can encourage behavior and decision making that is contrary to good patient care. The quality of the selection, credentialing, training, education, and ongoing working partnership with physicians and other providers is absolutely fundamental to the effectiveness of the capitation arrangement. Capitation can only be considered to be successful when it is consistently coupled with good, high-quality, and patient-oriented health care.

The Relationship That Is Established between the Provider and the Payer Is Fundamental to the Effectiveness of the Capitated Arrangement

Effective capitation requires that the payer and provider are committed to working together and have a basic interest in each other's success and survival in the arrangement. Antagonistic, highly competitive, or very distant and disinterested relationships are antithetical to the dynamics that are required to sustain and nourish capitation over a multiyear period. In today's turbulent environment, fraught with short-term financial pressures and growing mistrust, these fundamental relationships are more challenging to develop and maintain, but no less essential.

Assuming "Bad Risk" in a Capitated Population Is Nearly Always Fatal

No amount of exceptional care management is sufficient if the payer and provider have overlooked basic underwriting, selection, and benefit design tenets, leading to a population of members who have highly distorted risk and health care needs (adverse selection). Many frustrated providers have valiantly struggled to "manage their way" out of situations where the underlying risk is very poor. Payers, reluctant to acknowledge their own accountability related to the risk selection, point the providers toward their own inadequacies. Instead, the problems are so deep that a candid review of the risk arrangement and the population enrolled needs to be done so that special provisions can be made to work together to improve or eliminate the situation.

Preparing for Negotiation Is Essential To Obtaining a Successful Capitation Contract That Will Work for Years To Come

Providers with a successful track record with capitation are masters of preparation, carefully defining their needs, obtaining relevant data and actuarial support, developing detailed tables, and establishing contingencies. Capitation is complex and has a number of nuances that other forms of reimbursement do not have. Knowing those nuances is required, and they can be acquired from a number of sources including the payer, other providers with similar proposed capitation arrangements, actuaries, attorneys, consultants, and industry literature, among other sources. (See the Managed Care Resource Guide—Exhibits II–1 through II–7).

Focus on Capitation and Obtaining the Necessary Expertise To Succeed Leads to Success

Many providers, recognizing that capitation involves risk, decide to get involved in a "small way." They often then underinvest in resources, fail to gain any critical mass, create little push for changes in behavior, and maintain a pluralistic approach to the way they practice and provide care. Successful providers working with capitation are cautious, as they should be, but make a fundamental organizational commitment to working effectively with capitation, in whatever form. They recognize that critical mass is essential to gaining the full attention and commitment of the participants so that behavior is modified.

Related to Focus, Success with Capitation Requires Exceptional Problem-Solving Skills

Regardless of past success, the quality of the preparation, or any other factors, the turbulence in health care today inevitably creates problems in capitated arrangements. Adverse risk develops. Practice pattern changes don't take hold. New treatment patterns develop. Network or medical group expansion brings in new, unknown participants. Any of these and many other variables can and do develop, resulting in problems and challenges. Providers with clinical, administrative, and financial staff capable of delving into these problems, analyzing them effectively, and developing executable action plans are always ahead in the capitation arena. Too many providers fail to follow through in their analysis, despite making a number of correct assumptions about the source or cause of the problem initially. They follow that stage by venting their frustration toward the payer, practitioners within the group, and toward the situation, thereby failing to move the problem toward an active solution.

The Health of the Provider Organization Directly Impacts Its Ability To Take Action Related to Capitation Problems and To Follow Through on Its Plans for Implementing Support Systems

Capitation encourages and drives change in provider behavior. Inevitably, those changes create discomfort and conflict. Confrontation about key decisions, role definition, changes in clinical tradition, and economics are necessary and do occur. Many provider organizations avoid confronting issues until the problems reach a critical stage. Other providers confront colleagues too personally and emotionally, creating needless rifts in the organization. Providers working effectively with capitation possess experienced physician leaders and administrators, who interact regularly, ask questions, challenge assumptions respectfully, but clearly, and intervene in a personal and timely manner with colleagues. Those organizations are also aware of their "culture" and invest significant time in organizational planning and development.

Mastering Data and Information Management Creates the Basis for Both Initial and Ongoing Success in Working with Capitation

As mentioned above, capitation is often complex in its formulation. A number of variables influence how much care will be needed, when it will be needed, and in what form it will be delivered. Additionally, there are a number of contractual provisions that affect what is covered under capitation and what is not. Actuaries and other experienced health professionals develop "the numbers," but the work with numbers only begins there. It must extend, for the provider, into the initial analysis related to contract assessment and negotiation and with an effective capitation contract, through its operational life. Operating in capitation without a good, fundamental data and information reporting mechanism is like flying a plane with no visibility and the instruments functioning poorly. Inevitably, there will be a crash. Providers who successfully manage with capitation develop, purchase, or contract for a reliable information system. They identify the essential elements of that system at its core and focus there first, making sure that they have something that is sufficient but not too complex and cumbersome. They establish regular reporting and actively use ad hoc capabilities, and they utilize staff skilled in data manipulation, analysis, and reporting. The most effective providers have created teams of information, financial, administrative, and clinical staff who work together in the analysis of data on a regular basis, brainstorming on patterns detected, and proactive steps to be taken.

Administrative, Financial and Clinical Systems That Support Capitation Well Are Simple, User-Friendly, and Updated Regularly

The tendency in managed care generally is to obtain advanced software capabilities. This investment can pay off as providers grow into a system's capabilities. The problem that develops though is that providers overlook other "systems" related to routine data analysis, reconciliations, patient identification, case management, and retrospective review. Optimally, these small systems are linked together and integrated on a common platform, but many groups and networks have developed workable processes that function on a manual or stand-alone basis. The key is to develop, in a prioritized manner, a comprehensive set of tools and processes that will support the provider in working with capitation. It's particularly important to have "early warning" monitors that enable a quick response and further analysis to uncover problems and opportunities. Responding with urgency to key indicators is built upon effective systems.

The Size of the Provider Network or Group Influences the Likelihood of Capitation Gain in Today's Health Care Insurance World, Much of the Talk Is about Attaining Economies of Scale and Critical Mass That Will Change Market Forces

Clearly, there are benefits to being large. At the same time, large provider networks working with capitation have often proved to be unwieldy, unable to create the focus, flexibility, and accountability that are essential in capitated arrangements. On the other end of the spectrum, small groups or networks are unable to attract a sufficient member base or support the infrastructure necessary to manage capitation effectively. An optimally sized group of providers accepting capitation ranges from 6 to 20 practitioners. Many larger networks have addressed this issue by creating "pods" or "mini-IPAs" or by organizing capitation around specific geographic sites or specialties. Thereby, they gain the benefit of spreading the fixed cost of their infrastructure investments over a large base while establishing the peer accountability and focus of smaller units, at risk together.

LOOKING FORWARD

Health care, despite its turbulence and restructuring, continues to grow as an industry. As "baby boomers" age, the demand for health care services will continue to increase. Yet, the delivery of health care and our emphasis on health and wellness remains relatively unchanged. Structural and functional changes are required to create new emphases in health care that will facilitate improved health and better use of our resources. Capitation, in a variety of forms, is an economic tool or lever for that change. Economic incentives embodied in capitation do influence behavior. The challenge is to shape capitation to match the pace of market development and to enable providers to have positive experiences with it.

The future of capitation, though, is far from certain. Many still predict its demise. Others predict its proliferation. The reality, most likely, is that capitation will develop differently in each market. As other tools and approaches that lack economic incentives fail, though, the need for adapting and further developing capitation will increase. Underlying health care cost pressures, which lead to continuing price and premium increases, will force the reconsideration of the way providers are paid and therefore the way that they are involved in the redesign of the health care system.

Clearly, "consumerism" will support the market need for a variety of products, some of which are ill suited for capitation. As cost and premium pressures build, though, product and network design will develop increasingly around enabling new and more effective capitation arrangements. Moreover, the advances in information technology will support enhanced capitation management capabilities at a cost that does not require the large scale previously believed to be necessary. That is, smaller provider groups may well be able to utilize good information systems at an affordable cost. Finally, the continued growth in the supply of physicians, relative to their demand will create an interest and desire among younger physicians entering the industry to participate in these capitation arrangements. With the right pieces in place, as defined above, they will succeed, not only economically, but also more importantly, in reshaping the way that they think about and deliver their services to their patients and members. In the process, capitation will prove to be a powerful agent of change as we move into the twenty-first century.

PART II

Capitation Bootcamp

Day 1: Kinds of Capitation

Clifford R. Frank, MHSA

Today, managed care companies and providers often negotiate "capitation" as if there was only one kind of capitation. In reality, there is a spectrum of capitation and risk depending on the procedures and/or services included in the capitation agreement. This spectrum of risk and capitation level is best seen as follows:

The higher the number, the greater the risk (see Figure II–1). Let's look at each in more detail.

I. PRIMARY CARE ONLY

Primary care physicians (usually defined as Family Practice, Internal Medicine, Pediatrics, and often Ob/Gyn) are frequently presented with a "primary care only" deal. In this type of capitation, the primary care physician is obligated contractually to provide "typical" primary care services, usually those that are routinely offered in an office setting. It is critical that these services be defined by procedure code in the capitation contract, so there is no confusion as to what is included in the capitation. If possible, also have any limitations and exclusions defined clearly. In

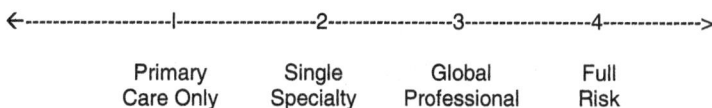

Figure II–1 Types of Capitation

addition, you must define who is responsible for out-of-area services to your members.

Primary care only deals are the least risky for the primary care physician since he or she generally has control over the utilization of primary care services. He or she can determine frequency of follow-up visits, use of typical primary care tests, etc., and can easily monitor such utilization on a patient-by-patient basis, thereby limiting his or her risk for unexpected high cost or high frequency procedures.

Usually, primary care only deals have some sort of "withhold" and/or "risk pool" arrangements. Withholds are designed to increase the primary care physician's risk and to provide an incentive to utilize a targeted amount of services and/or dollars. If he or she meets these goals, then the withhold is returned. Withholds are usually 15 to 20 percent of the capitation. If the withhold is higher, you need to know why and negotiate a more favorable rate.

Risk pools are often set up for Specialty Services and Inpatient Services. These are funded at predetermined levels using utilization and cost assumptions for the various services in the pool. If there is a surplus at the end of the year, the primary care physician and the MCO share in the surplus; if there is a deficit, plans vary, but some have the primary care physician and the MCO sharing in the deficit. Clearly, the primary care physician has a strong incentive to utilize only those specialty services and inpatient services that are absolutely necessary. The MCOs recognize this fact and most are very aggressive in monitoring quality assurance, profiling physician practices, etc., in order to not underutilize these services.

Primary care capitation figures vary depending on geographic area and lines of business, but are in the range of $10 to $13 per member per month for commercial business, $30 to $35 per member per month for Medicare business, and $8 to $12 per member per month for Medicaid business.

II. SINGLE SPECIALTY CAPITATION

In this form of capitation, physicians are capitated for their particular specialty. Common specialty caps are found in orthopedics, cardiology, mental health/substance abuse, ophthalmology, pathology, radiology, gynecology, urology, and dermatology. In single specialty caps, the primary care physician is not at financial risk, the respective specialists are.

Again, it is critical to know what is included in the capitation rate. The specialist needs to know if only the professional component is included, or if the institutional component is also included. Get inclusions in writing by procedure code if possible and get written exclusions and limitations.

Common capitation rates vary depending on specialty, but are usually between $.40 and $2.00 per member per month for commercial business. Medicare business should be around four to eight times the commercial rate, depending on the specialty (e.g., ophthalmology around eight times; mental health around one time; cardiology around five times; and gynecology around one time).

Since single specialty capitation rates are relatively small compared to the primary care capitation, it is important that the risk be spread over a sufficiently large number of members. In many cases, physicians are negotiating fee-for-service for the first 2,000 to 4,000 members, and then going capitation after they get enough volume to spread the risk.

III. GLOBAL PROFESSIONAL

Global professional capitation refers to full physician risk for all professional services—primary care and specialty care. Usually, covered services for primary care include internal medicine, pediatrics, family practice, routine lab and radiology, and general practice. Specialty care usually includes allergy, cardiology, dermatology, gynecology, mental health/substance abuse, neurology, obstetrics, physical therapy, emergency room, surgery, referral lab and radiology, pharmacy, and durable medical equipment.

Since most physicians can't control all of these medical services, the risk is substantially greater for any one physician. Global professional capitation is best done by large multispecialty group practices that can keep most of the services in-house and that can negotiate volume discounts as needed.

Commercial capitation rates should run two to two and one-half times the primary care capitation rate ($37 to $42 per member per month including primary care and specialty services). Medicare rates should be around three to four times the commercial rate.

IV. FULL RISK

Full risk capitation is just what the name implies; the contract is for all medical services—primary care, specialty care, and inpatient care (including deliveries, newborn care, room and board, and diagnostics). It is imperative that all covered services, including out-of-area emergencies, be defined clearly in writing. Limitations and exclusions also need to be clearly defined in writing.

At this point, the provider becomes a quasi-insurer and must have the infrastructure in place to manage care. This infrastructure includes some sort of eligibility checking, annual maximums, lifetime maximums, pre-authorization systems, concurrent review systems, and quality assurance systems. A good management information system is essential. Without one, don't even consider going full risk. Many MCOs may be willing and able to provide you with the needed infrastructure. In one case, the MCO installed a terminal in the provider's office and trained the office staff on how to check eligibility and maximums and enter pre-authorizations, all for no charge!

In full risk deals, the capitation rates are in the $80 to $90 per member per month range for commercial plans (excluding pharmacy) and $270 to $300 per member per month for Medicare plans, depending on the Adjusted Average Per Capita Cost (AAPCC). Pharmacy can run another $6 to $10 per member per month for commercial business and varies greatly for Medicare.

In short, not all capitation is the same. It varies by covered services and by level of risk. As more and more services are included in the capitation, the risk increases exponentially. Only providers with deep pockets, good MIS, comprehensive systems of care, and experience managed care staff should capitate the full risk deals being offered.

Day 2: How the Numbers Work—Capitation Calculations

Joel Hornberger, MHS

Many providers are afraid of capitation calculations, feeling that this "science" belongs to actuaries wearing black armbands and green eyeshades. Not true. Providers can calculate capitation rates and must understand the principles involved in capitation to protect their interests and to ask the right questions of the managed care entity. This section is written to show the practicing provider the basics of capitation, and the relative ease of calculating capitation (or analyzing the numbers presented to him or her) for a primary care practice and for a single specialty (in this case mental health).

THE BASIC CAPITATION FORMULA

Capitation = (annual utilization assumptions for covered procedures in "per 1,000 members") times (your costs or your charges per procedure) divided by 12 months divided by 1,000 members.

Here, capitation is expressed in dollars per member per month. Let's look at the numbers more closely.

Note that the capitation formula is based on *covered* procedures. These are the services for which you are contractually responsible, and they form the basis of your capitation. Different managed care organizations include different covered procedures, and you must know what procedures are to be included in the capitation rate. You need to get this in writing in the contract you sign with the managed care organization.

Conversely, you need to know what is specifically excluded from the capitation. Again, get it in writing *by procedure code* if possible. You need to see the "Group Master Contract" the managed care organization has with the employer, governmental agency, or other purchaser of its product. This will have the "Limitations and Exclusions" included in general terms, and you need to sit down with the managed care organization's provider relations staff and specifically define those procedures for which you are not responsible. (You also want to make sure you may provide these services on a fee-for-service basis and bill the patient, usually after informing the patient that the particular service is not covered by his or her insurance.)

The next critical numbers are the utilization rates for different procedures. These rate are usually expressed in "visits per 1,000 members," "procedures per 1,000 members," "days per 1,000 members," etc. Remember, these are *annualized* data. These are often tricky to find, but they can be found with a little work.

The best place to start is at your State Insurance Department (SID). The managed care organization is required by law to "file" its rates with the SID, and all rate filings are public information. Most often the rates are filed with specific "per member per month" or "per 1,000" details by various specialties, such as pediatrics, orthopedic surgery, mental health, etc. This is a gold mine of information since the managed care organization probably spent a lot of money to gather this information and file it. Get this information and compare it to the utilization they are using in their proposed capitation rate. You can tell immediately if (and how much) they are shaving off the rate they filed. Use the data to calculate your own rates as well.

If you've been practicing for any period of time, you know that different ages and different sexes use different amounts of medical services. As a result, the managed care organization may present you with several capitation rates, each for a different "age/sex" category. For example, there might be a rate of $2.87 per member per month for males aged 13–20, and a rate of $18.87 per member per month for females aged 25–35. In general, it is good to have age and sex adjusted capitation rates, but it makes your initial assessment of the rates more difficult (since you now have several rates to analyze and negotiate); and it makes the monthly reconciliation of your capitation check a nightmare since you will want to check the accuracy of your members' ages and sexes. If you have a large number of members (over 300 say), your risk should be spread sufficiently across the population so that you can use an "aggregate" capitation rate (the weighted average of the capitation rates for the anticipated ages and sexes).

The next numbers reflect your cost per service or charge per service. Many health care providers have trouble knowing their actual costs for performing certain services and prefer to use charges instead. If you calculate your capitation rate based on charges instead of costs, understand that the difference between the proposed capitation rate offered by the managed care organization and the capitation rate you calculate is your discount from charges. Don't forget to include additional overhead or administrative costs in your calculations. Most offices have found that managed care places a greater administrative burden on them, such that they often have to hire additional staff, install larger phone systems, buy computers, etc. Another big factor is the "hidden" cost of more physicians or other provider time dealing with utilization management, pre-authorizations, referrals, quality improvement, and other managed care details.

With the information above, you can now calculate a capitation rate. Since the numerator has "utilization per 1,000," you need to divide by 1,000 to get it to the "per member" level. Then, since the numerator is also

Table II–1 Capitation Case Study

CPT Codes In Capitation	Projected Annual Utilization/1,000 Members	Average Charge Per Service	(A x B)/12 PMPM
Office Visits	2.3	$ 50.00	$ 9.58
Inpatient, ER, Skilled Nursing Facility (SNF) Visits	0.2	$ 70.00	$ 1.16
Diagnostic/Preventive	0.4	$ 65.00	$ 2.16
Immunizations/Injections	0.3	$ 20.00	$ 0.50
Minor Office, Surgery	0.2	$ 30.00	$ 0.50
Minor Office, Lab	0.3	$ 12.00	$ 0.30
Other	0.1	$ 15.00	$ 0.13
		Total PCP Capitation before Adjustments	**$ 14.33**

Adjustment to Capitation (copayments)

Service(s) with Copayment	Projected Annual Utilization/1,000 Members	Average Collection Service	PMPM
Office Visits	2.3	$ 10.00	$ 1.92
		Total PCP Capitation with Adjustments	**$ 12.41**

Administration/UR/QA/etc. 10.00%			$ 1.24
		Total Capitation Plus Administration	**$ 13.65**

Table II–2 Mental Health Capitation Case Study

CPT Codes In Capitation	Projected Annual Utilization/1,000 Members	Average Charge Per Service	(A x B)/12 PMPM
Inpatient Days	30	$ 400.00	$ 1.00
Outpatient Visits	250	$ 70.00	$ 1.46
Detox Days	10	$ 300.00	$ .25
		Total PCP Capitation before Adjustments	$ 2.71

Adjustment to Capitation (copayments)

Service(s) with Copayment	Projected Annual Utilization/1000 Members	Average Collection Service	PMPM
Office Visits	250	$ 35.00	$ .73
		Total PCP Capitation with Adjustments	$ 1.98

Administration/UR/QA/etc. 10.00%			$ .20
		Total Capitation Plus Administration	$ 2.18

annualized data, you need to divide by 12 months to get "per month" figures. Therefore, you end up with dollars per member per month. (Some folks just divide by 12,000.)

After all this work, you're almost done. The number you have needs to be adjusted for the copayments you are due from your patients. These copayments usually are $5, $10, or $20 per visit, but can be as much as 50 percent copayment for certain types of services (usually mental health and substance abuse). You take the same utilization assumptions above and calculate the amount you expect to collect. Again, since these are in per 1,000 members per year, you need to divide by 1,000 and then by 12 (or just divide by 12,000 as a shortcut), to get "per member per month." Subtract this copayment number from your original capitation in order to get your final capitation.

Tables II–1 and II–2 are examples of a primary care capitation calculation and a single specialty capitation rate (in this case mental health and substance abuse). As you study these examples, remember the key steps to developing a capitation rate:

1. Know what's included in the rate (by procedure code).
2. Know what's excluded from the rate (by procedure code).

3. Obtain necessary utilization rates for the procedures, annualized per 1,000 members.
4. Obtain your costs or charges for the applicable procedures.
5. Multiply the utilization by the dollar figure.
6. Divide by 12,000 to get a "per member per month" rate.

Adjust the rate in the same way to account for cash collections due you from the patient.

Day 3: Bonus Structures under Capitation Contracts

Clifford R. Frank, MHSA

Nearly all capitation deals these days have some sort of bonus structure based on the physician's management of utilization. Whether you agree with these "incentives" or not, they are a part of capitation today and are likely to be a part of capitation in the future. Additionally, a lot of money is channeled through these structures, and they affect your bottom line. Here's how they work and what you need to look out for.

I. WITHHOLDS

Just as the name suggests, managed care plans withhold a specified percentage of your primary care capitation (usually 10 to 25 percent) and place these monies into an individual "withhold account." Theoretically, if you do a good job of controlling utilization and cost of service to members, you are rewarded by the return of your withhold money. If, on the other hand, you fail to meet certain utilization or cost goals, you lose that money. There are several key elements to watch in this arrangement.

First, your contract must be specific about the exact percentage of the capitation withhold. Surprisingly, some contracts are vague about the exact amount, or the amount of withhold increases during the contract period if utilization costs are higher than expected. This is particularly true in public systems, such as Medicaid HMOs.

Also, the withhold should be fixed for a specific time period, usually one contract period. Clearly, the smaller the withhold percentage, the less you are risking, so the more attractive the contract. Ask the managed care plan what percent of the withhold pools were returned over the past several years. If no one is getting the withhold back, then you can expect to lose yours as well, and there is a definite problem with the way the managed care plan is calculating the capitation or withhold. The product should be structured such that withholds are returned to high-quality, cost-effective physicians.

Second, your contract must clearly spell out how the remaining withhold money will be distributed. Generally, you should receive your withhold money within 60 to 90 days after the end of the managed care's operating year. To get your money this fast, the managed care plan has to estimate medical expenses that have been delivered, but that have not yet been paid. These are called IBNR (incurred but not received) claims.

Obviously, the managed care plan will estimate these IBNR claims conservatively, that is to their financial advantage, so make sure you understand how they are going to do the accounting. You can still protect yourself by negotiating for a "claims run off report" that will be done at a later date (after all claims are in and paid). This report will show the exact claims paid for the period, and monies may be due you at this time.

Third, if your withhold pool is going to be affected directly or indirectly by claims paid to referral specialists or inpatient providers, you should negotiate for the right to review specialist claims prior to payment by the managed care plan. Of course, this can be a time-consuming and tedious task, but can be immensely eye opening relative to fees being charged and procedures being performed. The managed care plan can't afford to get too far behind in their claims payment while you review them, so expect to negotiate some sort of required turnaround time.

II. RISK POOLS

Under most risk sharing plans, the managed care plan allocates a certain amount of money on a per member per month basis to various risk pools, often including a specialist pool and an institutional pool (see Figure II–2). When a claim arrives for one of your capitated patients for one of these services, it is paid out of the respective risk pool. At the end of the plan's fiscal year, account balances are calculated. If the money deposited into the various risk pools is greater than the money paid out, there is a surplus, in which you should share. If, on the other hand, the money deposited into the risk pools is less than the money paid out, there is a deficit. In this case, you need to know exactly what will happen, since you could end up having to pay money back to the managed care plan. This situation is especially galling when it is evident that the deficit is due to poor utilization management by the managed care plan.

Here are several things to watch when dealing with your risk pools.

Know the Contract Terms

The contract should state the mechanism by which a surplus or deficit is calculated, including use of IBNR and claims run off reports. The contract should also state exactly what will happen if there is a calculated surplus or worse, a deficit.

Know If the Amount Reserved in the Various Risk Pools Is Adequate

This is a difficult, if not impossible task, without incurring the cost of expensive actuaries. However, a quick estimate can be accomplished by

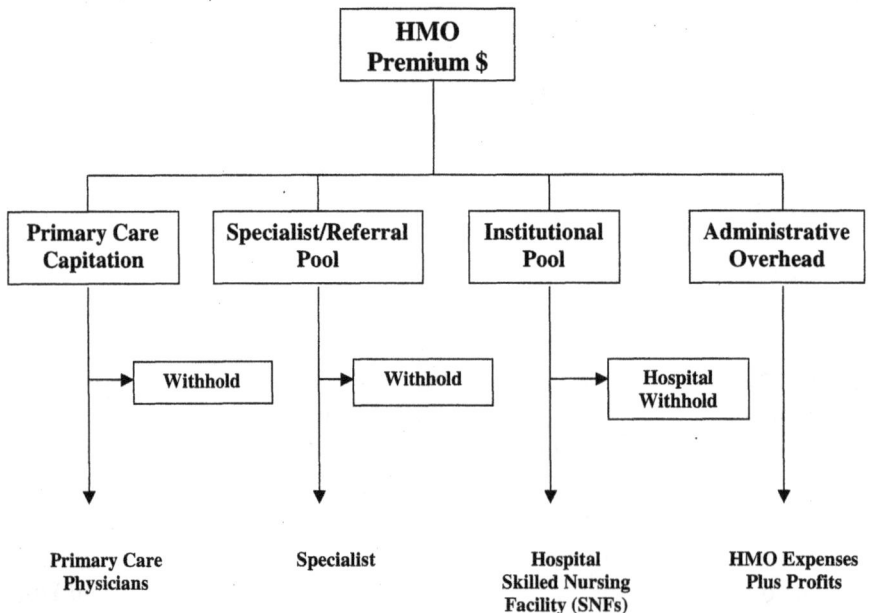

Figure II–2 Risk Pools

adding all the medical expenses (primary care capitation, specialist referral risk pool, institutional risk pool, and any other risk pools) and dividing
by the managed care plan's average premium. This should be at least 85 to
87 percent to ensure adequate risk pool funding. If the managed care plan
is unwilling to provide you with premium information, you can usually get
their rate filings from your State Insurance Department.

Know How the Surplus or Deficit Will Be Distributed

You should understand clearly when you will receive your money if
there is a surplus and when you will have to pay back money if there is a
deficit. Also, you need to know your maximum liability in the event of a
deficit. Try to limit your liability to 10 to 15 percent of the total capitated
payments made to you.

Know If You're in an Individual or Shared
Risk Pool

In an individual pool, you have total control. When you write a referral
or admit a patient, you know that those dollars are coming directly out of
your pocket. Clearly, this creates a strong incentive to control costs and
utilization. (Quality improvement plans and provider profiling are used to
monitor any abuses of the plan, including underutilization.) In a shared risk
pool, you are lumped in with everyone else who is writing referrals and
admitting patients. You have no control over their style of practice and,
therefore, can be hurt by overutilization from one of your colleagues. The
main advantage of the shared risk pool is the protection afforded by the
large numbers when all revenues and expenses are lumped together. Still,
many physicians are more confident in their own ability to manage costs
than in their colleagues' abilities, and prefer individual pools.

III. INVESTIGATE STOP-LOSS COVERAGE

Stop-loss coverage is used to insure against extreme liability resulting
from high overutilization or unexpected catastrophic expenses. Recently,
stop-loss coverage has become more readily available, although it may be

prohibitively expensive. However, it is worth investigating to protect you from unexpected losses.

Managed care plans are increasingly interested in "aligning" the financial incentives of the plan and the providers through a variety of bonus strategies. Those mentioned above are the primary mechanisms used, and new programs will certainly employ variations of these. Understanding withholds and risk pools is fundamental to success in managed care.

SUGGESTED READINGS

Incentive strategies reward winners, discourage sinners. 1998. *Capitation Management Report* 5, No. 11: 161–166.

One HMO's Physician Incentive Program Tries To Cover All the Bases. 1997. *St. Anthony's Physician Capitation Report*, July.

Pearson, S. et al. 1998. Ethical Guidelines for Physician Compensation Based on Capitation. *The New England Journal of Medicine* 339, No. 10.

Day 4: Physician Compensation Models under Capitation

Clifford R. Frank, MHSA

The good news is you got the capitation contract. The bad news is that if you conduct business as usual, the contract will kill you. Capitation payment changes incentives at the aggregate level. If your physician compensation systems do nothing to inject change into your physician compensation model, you may not be able to survive the resulting eventual financial disaster.

Capitated networks receive a flat monthly per member per month payment for a defined set of services, e.g., $1 per HMO member per month for all cardiology services. In such a case, a cardiology network may receive $60,000 per month to cover cardiology services for an HMO's 60,000 members in a defined geographic area. The issue is how funds should be split among the participating physicians in the network.

The first premise of physician compensation in capitation is that like should be grouped with like. This means that cardiologists and general surgeons should not share the same pool if possible. In a multispecialty capitation arrangement this premise means that the capitation should be subdivided into single specialty pools. Such dividing increases each specialist's impact on a given subpool and reduces the free rider problem of a few doctors not changing their high-utilizing practice patterns at the expense of everyone else. Free riders are more easily spotted when profiled against their specialty peers than when commingled with all physicians.

A problem with subdividing multispecialty capitation arrangements into specialty pools is the increasing statistical variation. Slicing pooled risk into thinner and thinner slices increases the impact of normal statistical volatility inherent in small populations. Having acknowledged that increased statistical variation, experience demonstrates that there is much greater value in increasing physician accountability by moving to single specialty targets. Statistical swings can be handled through stop-loss arrangements inside the global professional capitation, while still preserving the integrity of individual specialty risk pools.

Once the single specialty pmpm amounts have been established, disbursing funds among network participants can be a very divisive issue. Generally three approaches are available:

1. fee schedule with a withhold reserve against unexpected utilization
2. floating relative value scale
3. contact capitation—payment on a per patient basis

Using a fee schedule with a withhold requires physicians to accept a near-term reduction in payments for work they perform in the hope that if utilization is controlled, the withhold will be returned to each physician. If utilization is higher than targeted, then the withhold will be seized to pay the cost of the "overrun." The problem is that some physicians expect an "overrun," and they do not change their practice pattern. This results in those physicians receiving an undue share of the total compensation at the expense of their physician brethren. Their failure to control utilization usually results in fee schedule reductions or withhold increases over time.

Using a floating relative value scale involves paying out all funds each month without a withhold, but simply adjusting the payment rates each month to balance the work performed with the money available in the pool. One month the conversion factor may be .8 x Medicare, the next month 1.3 x Medicare, all depending upon the quantity of procedures performed in the month. Low utilization yields higher reimbursement to those who do procedures that month. High utilization means the unit value of each procedure is reduced. The problem with this method is that each physician is reduced to a market timer because if a physician turns his claims in on a light month, the rate is high. If it is a heavy month, the payment rate is low. This isn't utilization management; this is opportunism.

Both these modified fee-for-service disbursement methods for capitated contracts do not change incentives; they only introduce the concept of uncertainty on top of the concept of risk. These payment methods do not reward physicians for prudent decision making, except in the long term, and those incentives are weak behavior modifiers.

A third payment method, contact capitation, does gently affect incentives and enhances individual physician control over referral care.

Contact capitation pays physicians within a given specialty based on their pro rata share of patients managed. If a physician is managing the care for 12 percent of the patients in that specialty, then the physician will receive 12 percent of the capitation pool for that specialty that month. The next month, if the physician is managing the care for 9 percent of the patients in that specialty, then the physician will receive 9 percent of the capitation pool for that specialty that month. Each month the percent of patients being managed by each physician within the specialty is calculated, and money allocated on that basis. Patients are credited to a specific physician based on the initial patient contact (hence the name contact capitation) and are credited in that physician's panel for 12 months. A patient seen in March is credited in a physician's count in March and for 11 more months, regardless of how many times the patient is seen again. If the patient is seen in month 13, the process starts all over again for another 12 months.

Unlike a floating relative value scale or a fee schedule with a withhold, contact capitation moves some risk from the network down to the individual physician without unduly shifting so much risk as to burden the individual practitioner. Essentially contact capitation is a global fee per referral spread out over 12 months. Contact capitation changes incentives facing individual physicians. The physician must see the patient to obtain the first contact but has no additional incentive to put the patient through unnecessary visits, tests, procedures, or other costly interventions. The specialist physician under contact capitation must satisfy the primary care physician in his or her treatment of the patient, but if the specialist wants three or six visits to treat the case, the primary care physician no longer has to be the guardian of the visit bank. Under a contact capitation system, the flow between primary care physician and specialist is much smoother.

Contact capitation is complex to administer, and there are several modifications to the basic system that most specialties using contact capitation implement.

One modification is that certain procedures or diagnoses within a specialty may receive special consideration such as high-risk OB, AIDS, Whipple's disease, or other complex cases. In such cases, those referrals are usually specially weighted so as to fairly compensate practitioners who perform those procedures.

In other situations, capitated subpools may be created where complex cases can be identified, such as spine surgery, retina surgery, or other specialized procedures.

A third modification to the basic system is to reduce the time for a contact to count. In general surgery, most cases are resolved within 3 months so a 12-month contact window is unnecessary. A 3-month window is adequate for most situations. In radiology a one-month window might be sufficient.

Through the use of these modifications, most physician issues can be adequately resolved, but experience suggests that such modifications and resolutions are best reached by the physicians in that specialty themselves. Physicians within a specialty will deal with the "my patients are sicker" issue more effectively than administrators ever will. Implementing a contact capitation model is a difficult experience, but worthwhile over the long run because the incentives in the system become aligned throughout and because the process helps physicians communicate with each other about clinical effectiveness and outcomes. Particularly in chronic care, contact capitation rewards high-quality care, high-patient satisfaction, and good-patient outcomes, while keeping costs under control. A payment method that does all this deserves a look-see when it's time for you to capitate.

SUGGESTED READING

Pearson, S. et al. 1998. Ethical Guidelines for Physician Compensation Based on Capitation. *The New England Journal of Medicine* 339, No. 10.

Day 5: New Options for Aligned Payment Incentives among Specialists

Clifford R. Frank, MHSA

Contact capitation is an emerging payment system for specialty physicians involved in risk contracts. Contact capitation eliminates many of the problems associated with traditional capitation and offers the potential for both payers and practitioners to live with each other without combat. Contact capitation allows physicians to participate in the savings that they individually create in providing care more efficiently and effectively to their patients. It does not require a payer or network to severely restrict its physician panel in order to implement a risk-sharing model. As a consequence, payers and networks are looking to this reimbursement method as a means to containing their costs in the face of legislative and market demands for broader choice of specialists, direct or open access to certain specialties, and other new product designs.

The process of establishing contact capitation begins with the design of specialty risk pools. Creating these risk pools by specialty is necessary so that comparability among physicians is maintained. An underlying principle of contact capitation is that like should be pooled with like. A beginning point for that pooling is at the specialty level.

Creating specialty-specific pools requires either a significant amount of historical utilization data or access to external actuarial resources. In either case, the resulting analysis of the specialty pool data will result in an estimated per member per month expense for that specialty for each major product (e.g., Medicare HMO, commercial HMO). In addition, it may be necessary to develop specialty capitation rates by age segment, i.e., pediatric separate from adult. This may be necessary because different practitioners may be handling different age ranges of patients and will use services much differently.

A specialty pmpm capitation rate multiplied by the number of eligible members each month will create a specialty risk pool. The dollars in that risk pool must cover a contractually defined service mix that may include the following: professional services, office surgery and surgical tray, office medical supplies, injectables, inpatient professional services, outpatient surgical professional services, in-area non-network professional services, and office lab and x-ray services. The specialty capitation rate usually does not include the cost of implantable devices, facility inpatient and outpatient costs, diagnostic facility lab and x-ray costs, out-of-area costs, prescription drug costs, and services provided by other specialties that may include some of the same CPT codes.

Once a specialty capitation rate has been developed, the central issue remains as to how to split the risk pool funds among participating specialists. Usually one of three methods is used. First, a fee schedule with a withhold can be employed to disburse monies within the pool. This usually involves setting up a fee schedule that "should" be adequate to sustain the pool with budgeted utilization levels, and then withholding 20 percent as a reserve against utilization excesses. A second disbursement method often used is a floating fee schedule whereby the services performed each month are totaled and divided into the available risk pool monies. Funds are then distributed based on the resulting conversion factor and that conversion factor adjusts every month depending upon whether utilization is higher or lower than expected.

The problem with using fee-for-service methods to distribute monies inside a specialty risk pool is that the fee-for-service incentives remain in place, and the usual result is the risk pool runs out of money (and the network often blows up). With either fee-for-service disbursement method, an individual practitioner facing a set of treatment options that perhaps are marginal in benefit but substantial in revenue impact to his or her practice will face a strong incentive to continue to perform such procedures. In addition, to the extent that some physicians behave in a clinically conservative manner while others continue very aggressive treatment patterns, aggressive physicians are compensated for their work while conservative practitioners sacrifice revenue opportunities. In other words, the wild ways of some colleagues can destroy the economic underpinnings of the risk pool for the rest of the physicians in the network.

A third option is contact capitation. Contact capitation is a specialist physician payment system that pays physicians based upon the number of patients they manage within their specialty. Each month the specialty risk pool is allocated among the physicians in the specialty on the basis of the percentage of patients each specialist physician is managing, regardless of the number of procedures they perform.

A contact between a physician and a patient is established when the first patient visit occurs regardless of the location of service. That initial contact then credits the physician with a patient under his or her management for the next 12 months. At the close of each month, each physician's contacts are totaled and divided by the total number of contacts within the specialty. The specialty risk pool is allocated based upon each specialist's percentage of total patient contacts. For example, if the specialist has 9 percent of patient contacts in a particular month, then that specialist would receive 9 percent of the specialty risk pool. The next month, the same specialist might have 11 percent of active patient contacts, and that specialist would then receive 11 percent of the next month's specialty risk pool. Patients are credited to a specific physician based upon the initial patient contact. Those patients are counted in the physician's panel for the next 12 months. After the twelfth month, the patient is removed from the physician's count of contacts unless the patient is referred again by the primary care physician, in which case another 12 months of contacts are generated.

In most cases, contact capitation still requires an initial referral from the primary care physician. However, with contact capitation, the referral can function as a standing referral without the restrictions and limitation of many referral processes in place in managed care today. A primary care physician can simply note, "evaluate and treat" rather than limiting the number of visits, the conditions, or the scope of the referral to the specialist.

EQUITY ISSUES IN CONTACT CAPITATION

Internal specialty fairness is a major issue within contact capitation. Once resolved, fairness is also its strength. Because contacts can be adjusted for severity/complexity and other factors, and because physicians in that specialty usually make those adjustment decisions, the general perception of contact capitation is higher than other capitation payment models. When a physician presents an objection that his or her patients are sicker, several opportunities for making adjustments to contact capitation are available. First, the sickest patients or patients with particularly difficult diagnoses can be carved out from the contact capitation pool. On the other hand, another more common method is to weight those patient contacts in such a way as to make contact capitation fair to all specialists.

Adjustments to contacts can be handled through four mechanisms:

1. contact weights for certain procedures
2. contact weights for certain diagnoses
3. creation of subpools for selected procedures
4. fee-for-service carve-outs

These adjustment decisions are best left to the specialists in each community so as to design a system that is fair and takes into account each community's local practice patterns.

Contact weights can be applied to a diagnosis or to a procedure. For example, patients with certain diagnoses that are very complex to treat could result in contact values three times the standard contact weight for a given specialty. GYN Oncology patients are routinely weighted three-to-four times standard GYN patients. Similarly, leukemia patients are often weighted three-to-four times standard oncology patients. In other cases, certain procedures may involve such a significant effort that extra contact points might be warranted. A committee of network specialists for a specific community usually makes such weighting decisions.

In some cases, professional activity across a specialty varies substantially depending upon the area of professional interests a clinician pursues. For example, in ophthalmology the retina subspecialists maintain that the work they perform on patients is substantially different from the work of other ophthalmologists. To accommodate their equity considerations, contact capitated networks have created new subspecialty designations for physicians treating just retina patients. The result is two ophthalmology pools, one for general ophthalmology, and the other for retina. They are funded separately; they are administered separately; and they are created as two separate specialties for purposes of contact capitation. Subpool arrangements can also be used to differentiate physicians by clinical specialty area when physicians have different training and scope of practice within a specialty. For example, in cardiology, invasive cardiologists and clinical cardiologists may overlap in the services that they provide patients, but the majority of their services are different. Some networks have created subpool arrangements for invasive cardiology by identifying, by CPT code, which services are invasive cardiology as distinguished from clinical cardiology. Procedures for cardiac catheterizations, stents, nuclear cardiology, and other selected procedures are used to create one invasive cardiology risk pool, and all other cardiology services, including office visits, treadmills, stress tests, and other clinical services, are in the clinical cardiology pool. A particular specialist may be paid from both pools but for different types of services.

ADVANTAGES OF CONTACT CAPITATION

The advantages of contact capitation are that the network is financially stabilized; the individual physicians are incentivised to provide appropriate care; individual physicians are protected from potential utilization excesses by their colleagues; and the model allows for a broad physician specialty panel so as to make it attractive to payers, employers, and members. In developing contact capitation, the network can stop the losses associated with capitated contracts and can transfer the costs of the learning curve onto physicians who need to learn. Because contact capitation transfers the economic penalty associated with overutilization from the network to the individual physicians, physicians become acutely aware of their utilization patterns and any need to improve. Contact capitation can serve as a wake-up call to physicians whose practice patterns have been unchallenged or who have otherwise been unresponsive to quality improvement efforts within hospital facilities.

Other advantages of contact capitation come from the alignment of the financial and clinical interests of the parties. Physician interest in disease management increases; physician interest in patient compliance with medications increases; physician utilization of facilities tends to decrease as marginal cases are handled through other mechanisms; physician interest in looking at best practices in their specialty increases; and the door for product standardization within facilities is open wider.

DISADVANTAGES OF CONTACT CAPITATION

The disadvantages of contact capitation are that it is still capitation and it requires a mind shift away from a procedure-driven mentality. Even for those who benefit under a contact capitation payment method, the shift in focus from procedures to care management is a difficult one. However, unlike fee-for-service payment systems, physicians do not benefit economically by resisting care management, but instead benefit by innovating new care processes and approaches. Another hurdle for contact capitation is its administrative complexity. The concept is easy to understand but administratively complex because the process involves linking business together over time in order to count contacts. Most claim systems cannot administer a contact capitation payment methodology, but several add-on processing modules are available in the market today.

SUGGESTED READINGS

Contact capitation provides entry vehicle for specialty carve-out organization. 1998. *Capitation Management Report* 5, No. 5: 73–76.

Zero-based budgeting eases the transition to specialty capitation. 1999. *Capitation Management Report* 6, No. 2: 22–25.

Day 6: What It Takes To Make It under Capitation

Clifford R. Frank, MHSA

INTRODUCTION

Capitation as a payment mechanism necessarily reverses traditional incentives facing providers accustomed to fee-for-service reimbursement. But changes in the economic structure are relatively easy to anticipate compared to changes required in internal procedures within the provider's office and the hospital, among related specialists, ancillary providers, and the HMO itself. This article focuses on many of the subtle operational changes required to successfully operate in a capitated program.

INFORMATION—THE KEY TO SUCCESS

The biggest difference under capitation is the importance of information. Identifying that a patient is a capitated patient is critical to all downstream choices and events that occur in the care process. Registering, identifying, flagging, and monitoring these capitated patients are essential tasks, but ones usually performed by the lowest paid employees in the providers' office.

If a capitated patient is identified incorrectly, unnecessary referrals may be made, wrong physicians consulted, delays in results reporting accepted, and batteries of ancillary tests ordered. If the patient is known as capitated, referrals will be managed more carefully, only consulting physicians on the referral panel will be picked, follow-up on test results will be more aggressive, and tests will be staged in sequence rather than all at once. Each of these changes is the result of simply knowing the patient is capitated and the provider is at risk for the cost of care—either through the capitation, through a referral bonus pool, or both. Not only must your office know that the patient is a capitated one, but each contact point with you must know that as well. For example, if the patient ends up at the hospital, and the wrong physician is contacted, a whole trail of referrals and expenses may be generated—and charged against your capitation. If the hospital fails to identify the patient as a capitated one, and the discharge process lags, it is your bonus pool that suffers the cost of the extra hospital day.

Specialists too must understand if a patient is capitated, either for themselves or for their primary care referral source. In either case, resource consumption, referral authorization, ancillary testing, and treatment costs all are monitored by (and sometimes charged back to) the primary care physician. As a result, the primary care physician is more acutely aware of costs, ancillary test ordering patterns, and compliance with referral procedures by specialists. Specialists who blindly charge ahead without understanding that the patient is a capitated one, either for the specialist or for the primary care physician who referred the patient, risk incurring the wrath of the primary care physician who has to eat those costs inside a bonus pool.

THE TELEPHONE: HINDRANCE OR OPPORTUNITY?

The second biggest difference under capitation is the use of the telephone. In fee-for-service medicine, the telephone is the enemy. It is disruptive, intrusive, unending, and doesn't generate any revenue. Under capitation, the telephone becomes a provider's friend. The telephone allows a provider to handle some situations without an office visit, thereby reducing costs. The telephone allows the provider to intervene earlier in a disease process, thereby reducing costs and enhancing quality. The telephone interruptions are no longer intrusions, but are cost-saving opportunities. Outgoing telephone calls to check on patients, appropriately authorize medications, make referrals, and communicate lab results, all save money, and make time for other office-bound patients. Under capitation, the telephone creates opportunity gains instead of opportunity costs as happens in a fee-for-service environment.

COPING WITH RECORDKEEPING

The third biggest difference under capitation is the struggle of keeping it all straight. Contracting with 15–30 plans is headache enough. Now imagine that one-third are capitated and the rest are fee-for-service. The administrative headache of switching mindsets back and forth is unbearable for many. Some practices have moved to capitation for the bulk of their business. Others have tried to keep certain physicians within the group as primarily fee-for-service, while others take on the capitation programs.

Many practices have developed special coping tools, such as chart face sheets with helpful prompts for physicians. Such face sheets may include a cap/noncap designation, whether lab and x-ray can be performed in office, which outside ancillary service providers must be used, whether certain procedures are paid fee-for-service (even if the overall contract is capitated), and whether certain specialists must be used.

For hospitals, too, this administrative burden is difficult. One hospital, facing a myriad of plans, developed a directory of directories for the emergency room and nursing unit staff to use when trying to find a physician to consult. This directory is a giant cross-reference of who participates in which plans so that consults and referrals can get to the right place. Nonparticipating on-call physicians greatly appreciate not being called on cases where they would not otherwise get paid.

PHYSICIAN EXTENDERS

The last big difference under capitation is the use of physician extenders. Capitated physicians more readily see the economic benefit of using physician extenders in their practices than do their fee-for-service brethren. Under capitation, the physician extender can be used to protect the integrity of the physician's schedule, while still providing flexible service to patients, referring providers, and unanticipated patient demands. A physician extender can handle the overflow and work-ins for primary care physicians quite well.

In specialty practices, the patient education, monitoring, and motivation functions are often transferred to the physician extenders due to time and availability constraints placed on the physician. Where the providers are paid for prevention, these physician extenders pay for themselves through better-trained patients, fewer emergency room visits, and more effective patient education and motivation.

Capitation is a new ball game for most practitioners. Making it under capitation requires thinking differently about all aspects of your practice and those of your referral sources. Capitation requires linkages to systems of care that may not now exist. Building those linkages takes thought and care. But not building them can cost you money in extra expenses, missed opportunities, and disrupted schedules. Making it under capitation requires you to think about what is happening to a patient before he or she shows up for a visit, rather than after.

SUGGESTED READINGS

Conrad, D.A. et al. 1998. Primary Care Physician Compensation Method in Medical Groups: Does It Influence the Use and Cost of Health Services for Enrollees in Managed Care Organizations? *The Journal of the American Medical Association* 279: 853–856.

RVU costing model takes guesswork out of capitation. 1998. *Capitation Management Report* 5, No. 4: 49–54.

Day 7: Is Your PHO, IPA, MSO Underpowered?

Clifford R. Frank, MHSA

Physician Hospital Organizations (PHOs) that are built on the cheap can easily run into trouble as the administrative demands of the contracts the PHO negotiates outstrip the infrastructure capabilities of the organization. This article is designed to be an early warning to PHOs and their partners about the core administrative capabilities these organizations should have in order to manage risk-bearing contracts.

The costs of inadequate infrastructure are bad decisions—bad contracting decisions, bad medical management decisions, bad credentialing decisions, and bad bonus allocation decisions. Without good management data, the PHO must rely on payer-based information that is usually less timely, less accurate, and has less flexible reporting capabilities. PHOs that rely on a payer to manage a multimillion-dollar contract are asking for trouble in contract renegotiations. If the payer has their data and your data, guess who has the best data for the negotiation?

PHO INFRASTRUCTURE

Elements of a complete PHO infrastructure are outlined below. Some pieces can be contracted out to other entities, but these elements are present in most risk arrangements because experience has shown that they are necessary to make the numbers work.

Contracting

Recruits providers, is responsible for the credentialing and recredentialing processes, maintains provider network, provides ongoing service and provider education/ training.

- Provider relations staff
- Credentialing coordinator
- Credentialing of verification process and site visit capability
- Provider communications and inquiries
- Provider administrative manual
- Provider file maintenance

Medical Management

Supports/manages clinical quality improvement, coordinates delivery of services, monitors and tracks utilization.

- Referral authorization management process—paper, telephonic, or electronic
- Precertification process for selected diagnoses and procedures
- Preadmission, concurrent and retrospective review for inpatient stays
- After-hours assistance for emergency/urgent care
- Case management for large cases—links to reinsurance
- Disease management for classes of illnesses
- Physician profiling and reporting
- Referral care protocols
- Medical necessity determination
- Medical appeals process

Claims Administration

Responsible for the general management and administration of claims processing functions and all related systems support.

- Provider file setup and maintenance
- Benefit adjudication table setup and maintenance
- Eligibility and enrollment database maintenance and reporting
- Eligibility verification and notification process

- Coordination of Benefits (COB) and subrogation management
- Physician change notification procedure
- Claims submission guidelines and procedures
- Guidelines for payment of non-network claims—authorized and un-authorized
- Claims data entry, adjudication, explanation of payment
- Check writing
- Activity reporting

Accounting and Financial Reporting

Administration and management of all accounting and financial activity including financial reports and analyses, maintenance of accounting systems.

- Set up pools for each risk category
- Charge network claims against correct pool
- Charge non-network claims against correct pool
- Track large claims against reinsurance attachment points
- Generate financial statements including IBNR claims lag
- Generate bonus pool reports
- Disburse bonus checks, if any
- Generate 1099 reporting
- Generate reinsurance reporting

Payer Contract Compliance

Monitor contract guidelines/terms and provide contract analysis to assist with contract negotiations.

- Minimum premium guarantees
- Transfer cases
- Carve-outs, supplemental payments
- Late enrollees

- Underwriting guideline compliance
- Product mix/risk mix changes

Member Services

Provide members assistance with enrollment process and routinely interact with members by providing ongoing customer service.

- New member orientation
- ID card generation/verification/oversight
- Physician selection/change
- Appointment assistance
- Administrative advocacy
- Benefit coverage information
- Member inquiries

Information Services

Maintain information systems, provide data management, and provide systems analysis to enhance data and reporting capabilities.

- Eligibility interfaces with payers
- Database administration/maintenance
- Provider/Payer/Member/Employer/Procedure/Diagnosis file creation and update
- Link medical management decisions to payment process, provider file, and credentialing
- Multiple reimbursement methods by provider
- Claims payment interface with payers
- Bonus calculation—deficit/surplus carry-forward

The functions described above are often handled by payers for their own business. A PHO will be handling many of these functions for several payers, thereby making the process a complex one. One of the allures of PHOs is that they will standardize procedures so that all payers accessing the PHO will do things the same way. Rarely is that end accomplished fully. But standardization can be more likely achieved if payers delegate these functions to the PHO. For delegation to occur, payers must be assured that the PHO can effectively assume responsibility and deliver on those promises of administrative performance.

If payers delegate certain functions to the PHO, then the process the PHO uses becomes a standard one for all payers. Thus, if referral management is delegated, then primary care physicians use one form, one set of referral criteria, one phone number, and one referral specialist panel. If some payers refuse delegation of referral management, then the PHO needs to guide its physicians through several referral processes, which diminishes the attractiveness of the PHO to physicians.

PHOs that started as contracting organizations and are now ready for more will find payers resistant to delegating certain important functions unless the infrastructure is present within the PHO. Such infrastructure carries with it costs in terms of people, computer systems, phone systems, and space that somewhat duplicate structures already present at payers. Only when the processes are standardized across numerous payers will savings offset the expenses incurred in infrastructure costs. But these investments pay off in other ways through utilization savings bonuses, better decisions, quicker analyses, and enhanced provider control of clinical and administrative processes. Such intangibles are valuable to professionals who cherish their autonomy and accept accountability through risk contracts.

SUGGESTED READINGS

Peters, J. 1999. Turning Around a Troubled MSO: A Strategic Approach. *Health Care Strategic Management* 17, No. 1: 1, 20–23.

Use caution before taking on claims processing. 1998. *Public Sector Contracting Report* 4, No. 5: 65–70.

Day 8: Is Your Practice Management System Ready for Capitation?

Clifford R. Frank, MHSA

Capitation deals present huge challenges to practice management systems. Fundamental changes must occur in the practice management system as health care delivery moves from fee-for-service reimbursement to capitation arrangements.

The greatest challenge to a practice management system is that it must now become a risk management tool rather than a simple billing and accounting tool. Many organizations fail to understand the difference and enter into capitation deals without the information system to support them. The following are capitation system requirements that provide a tool for organizations to assess future practice management systems, communicate with consultants or systems developers on their needs, or analyze their own system's capabilities to handle capitation deals. Remember, managing your risk is the name of the game in capitation, and your system must do that.

SYSTEM FUNCTIONALITY REQUIREMENTS

Membership and Eligibility Capabilities

In capitation management, you can't afford to provide services to ineligible members. You are receiving a certain amount of money "per member per month." Members are assigned to you, and it is your job to provide care for them according to the covered services defined in your contract. If you are providing services to ineligible members, you are not only losing your pmpm money; you're also losing possible fee-for-service revenue billable to the patient or to another third party. Your computer system must have the capability of maintaining complete demographic data for all your assigned members. Ideally, it should also include data on current benefits (including covered services), member copayments, and historical information about the members' prior coverage and PCP assignment.

Your member data needs to be accurate and timely so you can always tell who's covered, who's not, and track eligible members with confidence.

Ideally, your system should be able to:

- automatically verify member eligibility
- automatically verify member benefit coverage for requested services
- automatically verify member year-to-date and lifetime-to-date benefits
- identify possible COB coverage(s)

Benefit Plan Management

Your information system must be able to easily and accurately track various benefit plans and link them to specific members. Just as you can't afford to provide care to ineligible members, you can't afford to provide noncovered services to eligible members. One health care provider didn't know that Attention Deficit Disorder (ADD) was a noncovered service under a certain HMO plan and provided over $70,000 of ADD care, only to be told that the service was not covered. Your cap deal will specify in the contract which benefits are covered and which are your responsibility within your capitation rate. These should be listed by procedure code, diagnosis, or revenue code. Your system must be able to tell you and your other practitioners what services are covered at the procedure code level. It should also be able to monitor and "catch" authorizations, referrals, or payments beyond an eligible member's benefit level.

Your system should be able to:

- automatically verify covered benefits at the procedure code level
- automatically verify excluded benefits at the procedure code level
- link covered benefits to authorizations, referrals, etc.

- link covered benefits to your internal utilization management system
- link covered benefits to your internal quality assurance system

Provider Payment Mechanisms

Your system absolutely must be able to provide flexible provider compensation. The variety of cap deals out there will cause you make some tough compensation decisions, and you need the reimbursement flexibility to align everyone's financial incentives. Contact capitation is the latest, and some say the best, method of funds distribution. Your system, however, also needs to be able to work with withholds, bonuses, relative value units, Resource Based Relative Value Scale (RBRVS), fixed fee pmpm, percent of premium, percent of charges, etc. If your system is weak in this area, your risk increases dramatically, and provider satisfaction decreases dramatically. In other words, you're in trouble. Reimbursement calculations must be done quickly, accurately, and timely. Ideally, this system communicates with your payroll or AP system.

Your system needs to:

- handle a variety of ways of paying physicians
- be able to link to patient satisfaction measures and pay accordingly
- distinguish physician quality/performance measure and pay accordingly

Internal Utilization Management

Now that you're capitated, you have to manage your own risk. With capitation, you have a lot more freedom to practice the way you want, but with that freedom comes the opportunity to overutilize or underutilize care. Your system must be able to track the utilization of health care resources used to treat eligible members. You must monitor and/or perform referral tracking, encounter tracking, and specialist or consultant tracking. Your system must be able to track inpatient admissions, lengths of stay, and continued stay reviews. Utilization appropriateness determinations are now your responsibility under capitation, and you must be able to track them. Your system must be able to combine individual care resources into complete episodes of care in order to capture "input" resources per member or per case.

Your system needs to:

- generate authorizations or referrals by procedure, diagnosis, place of service, etc.
- override authorizations based on user-defined criteria
- provide open file space for "notes" for each authorization
- track episodes of care and, ideally, monitor outcomes

Medical History Database

Capitation changes everything, and one thing it especially changes is disease management. Your system needs to be able to provide information on the complete continuum of clinical information, not just individual services. It must also be able to detail each service encounter across the continuum of care. You must be able to set up quality indicators and use your system to measure them. This is particularly important when negotiating contracts since you need to be able to "prove" quality.

One of the biggest challenges to your system is the measurement of medical outcomes. Increasingly, managed care companies are becoming accredited by the National Committee for Quality Assurance (NCQA), and outcomes is an expanding area of concern within NCQA. Also, payers (and especially self-funded employers) are asking the question, "What am I buying with the millions of dollars I'm spending on health care?" You need to be able to answer that question with a solid medical database that can measure outcomes for their covered lives.

Finally, you need to be able to profile providers, so you can see the various medical inputs by provider and the resulting health outcomes. This is an invaluable tool in helping to manage capitation risk and is powerful when physicians see how they compare to their peers.

Your system needs to:

- detail episodes of care
- identify health care outcomes
- compare your outcomes to others, e.g., community or epidemiological data

- profile providers based on medial inputs and health outputs
- "prove" quality

Financial Requirements

Usually, practice management systems are strong in this area. However, capitation forces a system to account differently, especially if you are capped and are paying out-of-your-network claims. Ideally, your system should be able to distinguish key contract terms and conditions and, essentially, be a contract management tool. It should also be a contract simulation tool, complete with your proprietary database (mentioned above), so you can analyze proposed capitation deals.

If you are paying claims, your system needs to be very sophisticated in terms of automatic verification of members, covered services, copayments, coding, payee, authorization verification, fee schedules, possible COB, ability to capture all HCFA 1500 and UB92 fields, and historical lifetime or annual limits. Some practices use their regular Accounts Payable system to pay claims; this is a mistake since AP systems do not capture the data you need to manage your risk. (Important Note: Don't pay claims unless you have to! Use a third-party administrator (TPA) and let them have the headaches. It's worth the money.)

Your system should also let you do copayment billing of members. It should let you track your stop-loss coverage (both specific and aggregate); as well as let you do risk pool accounting. Your system must be able to track out-of-network or specialty charges. (Some global cap deals place you at risk for inpatient, specialty, lab, radiology, etc. and you need to track all these.)

Of course, your standard financial functions such as billing and collections, production of financial statements, budget formation, accounts receivables (AR), accounts payables (AP), general ledger (GL), etc., are all fundamental components of a good capitation financial system.

Your financial system needs to:

- track stop-loss
- perform reimbursement calculations
- manage contracts

- pay claims (if necessary)
- handle traditional financial functions
- simulate capitation deals

Report Generation

In capitation, your risk management is only as good as your information. You need accurate reports, usually in a hurry. Your system should have predefined or customized reports.

At a minimum, your system should provide you with:

- eligibility listings
- pmpm calculations (costs)
- authorized services
- utilization reports
- provider profiles and reports
- encounter reports
- outcomes
- disease management indicators
- clinical pathways
- utilization management reports
- cost accounting reports
- stop-loss accounting reports
- case mix data

Capitation contracts require a new way of doing business, and your information system is at the center of health care revolution. If it is able to handle the complexities of this revolution, you're on your way to a bright future in the "new-world." If it's not, well . . .

SUGGESTED READING

Look beyond the sales pitch when evaluating capitation IS. 1999. *Capitation Management Report* 6, No. 4: 49–53.

Day 9: Capitation Pitfalls To Avoid

Clifford R. Frank, MHSA

Capitation programs are full of potential pitfalls, both for you and the HMO. An essential ingredient to capitated contracts is a willingness to make things work. But, some situations are beyond immediate resolution. And, it is those situations that will tax the good will of all parties. You can avoid some of these pitfalls by thinking through and discussing the "what ifs" with the HMO in the negotiation process. Here are 10 surprises that others have found out about the hard way.

Patient Identification Problems

If the patient is not identified as a capitated patient by all providers in the network, somewhere along the line a problem will develop. The wrong specialist will be consulted; the wrong lab will be used; the sense of urgency will be missing; and, even a different clinical path may be followed. The HMO must educate all its providers that certain subspecialties are now capitated, certain hospitals have capitated arrangements for specific groups, and primary care physicians must explicitly authorize referrals to noncapitated specialists. If the hospital fails to contact the right consulting physician, who pays? If a primary care physician refers a patient to a noncapitated specialist, who pays? If the patient fails to inform the hospital or physician of his or her HMO coverage for several days or treatments, what happens? This is a problem particularly for Medicare HMOs where seniors present their Medicare card rather than their HMO card or where a clerk has recorded the Medicare HMO as a Medicare supplement policy.

Calling the Wrong Specialist

This happens often if the patient is not identified as a capitated patient. But it can happen many other ways as well. If the hospital has an EKG reader panel, and you are a capitated cardiologist, how is the hospital going to get your capitated patient's EKG to you instead of to the EKG reader panel? If they don't, who pays the EKG reader's bill? Patients in the emergency room present another nightmare. You are not on call, and a non-network physician is consulted by the emergency room. Who pays? At what rate? What if that physician authorizes admission, and you would not have done so? Who pays?

In-Area Emergency Risk

Everyone knows to toss out-of-area risk out of the capitation contract. But the greater risk lies in in-area risk. It happens more often, and results in more confusion. Transfers to your facility are less likely because the patient is most likely on his or her way home by the time you find out about it. Who authorizes care? Who pays? At what rate? Under what circumstances?

DEDUCTIONS FROM CAPITATION

This is the "gotcha" section of most capitation contracts. It looks harmless but is loaded with danger. The mechanics for deducting funds from your capitation often govern how the issues noted above are settled. If deductions unilaterally occur by the HMO, your opportunity to approve/deny, insist on adequate documentation, and actively intervene in costly situations will be limited. The HMO will not be well motivated to intervene in difficult situations on your behalf, because the HMO will simply deduct the cost of the errant referral, admission, or visit from your capitation. If, on the other hand, the provider first approves all deductions, then the burden of proof is on the HMO as to why something should be charged against your capitation fund.

Overlapping Service Capabilities

You are a capitated cardiologist. You have certain cardiac stress testing equipment in your office, and such tests are included in your capitation. But the hospital also has such equipment. How are those capitated patients who show up at the hospital for stress tests going to be turned away? Who pays for their stress test if the hospital fails to turn the patient back to your office? What about a general internist who is primary for some of these HMO patients who also performs stress tests? Who pays him or her? Who tells him or her not to do that anymore? Who makes your referral source mad?

Patient Punting

When a capitation program is put in place, patients with multiple problems become problem patients. Physicians have been known to turf patients to other physicians for treatment of their other ailments first. Also, capitated primary care physicians may turf cases they used to handle once they find a capitated specialist to handle them. If no additional charges are applied to the primary care physician's referral pool for referring to capitated physicians, the referral rate can be expected to jump. Who monitors such situations? Who sanctions such behavior? What behavior constitutes dumping? How does the Medical Director of the HMO actually intervene? Does the HMO really develop referral protocols as they say they will or have? Have you seen them? Who enforces them?

Who's In, Who's Out—Who Decides?

Forming specialty networks is tricky business for providers. Yet letting the HMO form them may result in fragmentation of your business or worse. For specialty capitation, picking the right physicians is essential, but "right" from whose perspective? What if you pick a specialist you respect, but the primary care physician's feel is unresponsive? What if the primary care physicians like two-thirds of your specialty group, but not the rest? What do you do? What if not all of your network can handle capitation equally well, who decides who goes? What role does the HMO play in making any or all of these decisions?

Who Else in the Network Is Capitated, Now or in the Future?

Think of the plight of the capitated physical therapist if the orthopedists were not capitated when the physical therapy deal was originally cut. What happens to the physical therapist if the HMO institutes an orthopedic capitation? PT volume doubles while the capitation remains fixed. Understand the capitation context completely before you do a deal and leave "wiggle-room" in the contract if the context changes.

Risk Selection

The HMO has enrolled a mix of both high- and low-utilizers. If the HMO sells a large high-utilizing group like a school district, the capitated providers are going to take a hit. The HMO's sales strategy and enrollment targets directly impact the capitated provider. HMOs will not turn over control of their marketing program to capitated providers. They will, however, share their current demographic makeup including major industrial groupings, age and sex distribution, and geographic distribution of their membership. This information may be helpful in anticipating utilization surges.

Who Collects and Manages Data?

Under capitation, with data comes control. If you are depending on the HMO for utilization and financial data, you are destined to have an expensive lesson in the power of information. Reports will be generated to meet the HMO's needs, not yours. Analysis of the data will require "special runs" and will either cost extra, take six months, or both. If you are trying to manage care without aggregate data or comparative data, you are reduced to playing cop on a case-by-case basis. This sounds a lot like what the HMOs do now. Do you want to do to others what they do to you? Or do you want to assemble information in a way that is meaningful to you to make better clinical decisions?

Day 10: Minimizing Risk When You Capitate

Clifford R. Frank, MHSA

INTRODUCTION

Although several capitation deals may land on your desk in a given week, not all deals are alike, even if the capitation rates are. Minimizing your financial exposure while maximizing your upside potential in these arrangements is the goal. Here we present several techniques for protecting yourself.

CAPITATION COMFORT ZONE

First, try to take risk for only those services that you provide. If your scope of practice is narrower than what the standard contract provides, you would be better off taking a lower capitation rate and referring out those other services than forcibly expanding your services beyond your comfort zone. Similarly, if the capitation is for specialty services or hospital services that your network does not provide, subcapitate to another network or facility if possible. Don't take risk for things you or your network doesn't do.

Second, try to get the capitation age/sex adjusted. This is especially important in primary care. Utilization varies greatly based on the age and sex of the patient mix. If the deal is a flat rate, you may end up with a mix of patients older and more female than otherwise anticipated in the capitation rate development formula. By getting the capitation age/sex adjusted, you get more money if your mix is skewed toward heavily using populations.

Third, make sure you get an adequate number of members with which to spread the risk. Some plans capitate primary care physicians from the first patient. Others will wait until you have a base of 50 or 100 patients. The second method is preferable because one sick patient can really destroy your capitation pool. Primary care capitation only really works if you let the law of large numbers work for you. This means you really have to jump in. You can't do it just a little bit because you will most likely get burned.

CHECK OUT ENROLLMENT MATERIALS

As part of the enrollment process, check your listing in the HMO's provider directory it hands out to new members. This is most likely the only information people will have to select you or someone else. Make sure you are listed in the primary care section if you are primary care. Make sure the listing is correct and complete. If you have extended office hours, get the word out to the HMO's enrollment clerks. People will choose such offices even if they don't intend on using the extended hours, just because they think they might want to sometime. If you are a specialist who wins primary care, watch out. You will likely attract patients who know you and love you and who are sick as anything. They will lovingly bankrupt your capitation pool and if you don't have enough new healthy patients to offset their higher utilization, you will lose money.

PROVIDER STOP-LOSS

Fourth, provider reinsurance or stop-loss is another program you may look into. Many HMOs offer reinsurance to hospitals for claims above a set dollar threshold. For example, the hospital may receive from the HMO $800 per day unless the case exceeds $40,000—in which case the hospital receives 70 percent of its charges. This prevents the hospital from facing an economic disaster if a patient incurs several hundred thousand dollars of charges on a 45-day stay. Such reinsurance is often available for capitated providers to purchase, either through the HMO or through a commercial reinsurance broker. These products are complicated and filled with little loopholes, so be very careful to discuss the arrangement thoroughly with a knowledgeable financial advisor. In general, however, having reinsurance is a good idea if you have a small number of patients, or your finances can't take the impact of a major claim, should one occur.

BONUS POOLS

Fifth, make sure the HMO adequately funds the bonus pools. If the pools are underfunded, then you will not likely get much of a utilization savings bonus at the end of the reporting period.

An example looks like this: HMO "A" has a primary care capitation contract that pays $12 per member per month plus a bonus of 25 percent of the hospital risk pool if utilization is favorable. So far, so good. But, what are the hospital utilization targets? They won't tell you if you don't ask—so ask.

Let's assume HMO "A" says 280 hospital days per 1,000 enrollees per year. Ask them what their hospital utilization is running currently. HMO "A" has bounced around 260–300 hospital days per 1,000 enrollees for the last year and a half. Therefore, 280 days doesn't look like too good a target. Odds are the plan won't hit it, and you won't get your bonus. But wait, it gets worse. Let's further assume that HMO "A" funds its hospital bonus pool at $750 per hospital day. But you know their cost at your hospital is $800 a day.

Ask the HMO how their actual cost per day compares to their formula cost per day. If actual is greater or even close to formula, the bonus fund won't cover the actual utilization, and there will be no bonus. The funding formulas can be renegotiated if the HMO really wants you as a primary care physician. However, you have to ask for the information, evaluate it, and insist on either changes to the formula, or at least a fresh look midway through the bonus period.

Minimizing risk in capitation deals can be accomplished through careful analysis of the financial arrangements. But it also requires a genuine spirit of cooperation from the HMO to really be effective. Only you can evaluate on that spirit on a case-by-case basis, but they all will say they want to be your partner. Choose carefully, but not timidly.

SUGGESTED READINGS

Anderson, G. and Weller, W. 1999. Methods of Reducing the Financial Risk of Physicians under Capitation. *The Journal of the American Medical Association* 8: 149–155.

Can providers survive when accepting pharmacy risk? 1999. *Capitation Management Report* 6, No. 3: 33–36.

Get Plans To Pay for New Drugs and Technologies. 1999. *Managed Care Contract Negotiator*, February.

Day 11: Coverage Definitions Affect Capitation

Clifford R. Frank MHSA

Coverage definitions can trap providers into covered service they did not intend, nor, in many cases, control. Any capitation deal can work if the basket of covered services is defined right. If the capitation looks low, carve out a few more services. Of course, the HMOs understand this logic, too. In fact, they have better data than do providers, so HMOs know exactly the value of each carve-out.

PLAN DESIGN

Plan design is a hidden trap that most providers overlook. If a Medicare HMO provides drug coverage at a level substantially higher than its competitors, and you are considering a capitation for this HMO—watch out! The likely health status of the HMO's enrollees will be lower, and their costs higher because of the richer drug coverage benefit. If the enrollees are sicker, but the capitation rate is not enriched, the provider takes the hit. You pay for the HMO's bad benefit design.

IN-AREA EMERGENCY ISSUES

In-area emergency care is a big hole. Providers understand the necessity for eliminating out-of-area coverage from their capitated liability. But in-area emergency sounds more reasonable. It isn't. If you are a capitated provider for specialty services and a patient seeks care at a hospital emergency room where you are not on staff, anything goes. A network physician may or may not be called in on the case. The HMO may or may not be notified. You may or may not receive a transfer. But, you will get the bill if in-area emergency care was not specifically excluded from your capitation agreement. Even if the facility is one in which you routinely practice, the emergency room or staff nurse may contact the on-call physician rather than your capitated group for a patient requiring medical services. You'll get the bill for that one, too, if you haven't negotiated the deal carefully.

MEDICAL NECESSITY

Medical necessity determinations are another trap. If the HMO is capitating providers, the HMO often is implicitly turning over medical necessity determinations to the capitated providers as well. Since these providers usually do not have the same insulation from their colleagues as an HMO Medical Director, the result can be far fewer medical necessity denials. While this may seem a happy result of capitating providers, the effect is to lower your pay. Capitated providers are the ones bearing the cost of the increased utilization (due to fewer denials) but without additional revenue to offset the utilization expense.

OVERLAPPING SERVICES

Services that overlap among providers create several benefit and capitation computation problems. For example, if you are a capitated general surgeon, carpal tunnel surgeries fit under your jurisdiction. However, they can be performed by neurosurgeons, orthopedists, and general surgeons. What happens if all the carpal tunnel cases now end up in your office instead of split among the three groups? This situation could happen if the primary care physicians have a referral pool bonus, and the other surgical specialties are still fee-for-service.

Services that overlap between professional and institutional providers can cause problems as well. Cardiac testing performed in the office may be capitated, but if cardiac testing at hospital-based programs is also capitated inside the cardiology capitation, there will be some big problems. Office lab and x-ray pose similar problems if not spelled out clearly. Further, sometimes spelling it out isn't enough if the HMO's computer system can't handle the administration of the definition. Or worse, your front office staff can't effectively route the right patients to the hospital for testing and others to your office-based diagnostic testing center.

INCENTIVE PROGRAMS

Coverage definitions are just as important to review when looking at incentive programs within the capitation arrangement. When an HMO is offering incentives based on certain utilization targets being obtained, make sure the definitions of those targets are well understood. For example, if the target is 240 hospital days per 1,000 people per year, what constitutes a hospital day? Do observation days count as a hospital day? What about newborn baby days? Do mental health days count the same as medical/surgical days?

CAPITATION CARVE-OUTS

Carving out high-cost, low-frequency services is a generally well-understood method of lowering risk in capitation programs. For primary care physicians, common carve-outs involve immunizations, well-woman exams, flexible sigmoidoscopies, and inpatient services. For specialists, carve-outs may include procedures or diagnoses that involve costly equipment or supplies, many ongoing visits, or cases that usually involve multisystem failure. Carve-outs can be on a procedure code or diagnosis code basis, or some combination of the two.

DETERMINING ELIGIBLES

Determining eligible members is another ongoing headache. The HMO enrolls the member and pays the provider the negotiated capitation rate. However, if the HMO is slow to tell the provider of added members (and additional revenue), the member may present without the provider being aware the patient is a capitated member. Worse, the member may be presenting at a specialist's office without a referral, for a capitated service. Depending on the wording of the hold harmless clause, you may not be able to bill the member for that visit because the HMO failed to notify you of the member's status. Terminated members are another problem. If the HMO fails to notify the provider that a member has terminated, you may continue to see the member unaware that you have not been, and likely will not be, paid.

HMO programs come and go. But understanding what you have bought, or what you have been stuck with, is important to making it work. Generally, the more complicated the mechanics of the program are, the more likely it will blow up, because the risks and the rewards will end up in different pockets.

SUGGESTED READING

Get Capitation Fees for New Plan Members before They Get Sick. 1997. *Managed Care Contract Negotiator*, December.

Day 12: Contract Provisions To Avoid

Clifford R. Frank, MHSA

INTRODUCTION

When physicians and administrators think of "risk" in managed care, they often think of capitation, withholds, and risk pools. This "financial fixation" causes many providers to overlook nonfinancial contract provisions that create tremendous risk for them. These are 10 key contract provisions that, if negotiated properly, can help reduce risk.

Definitions

Most managed care contracts have a section on definitions and most providers read these definitions quickly, in order to move on to the more interesting financial sections of the contract. Big mistake. Read each definition carefully and be prepared to ask questions if you don't understand it. Many definitions in managed care contracts are incomprehensible or just plain sloppy. The following is an actual contract definition:

> Capitation Payment: Means the payment paid to the Provider as the projected cost of all Primary Care Services covered under a Health Services Agreement which a Member in a specific payment category is expected to use during a month's time.

This "definition" fails to identify when the capitation payment is due, the CPT codes included in "Primary Care Services," what the "Health Services Agreement" actually is, and what constitutes a "specific payment category." It is vague, misleading, and confusing; and if the time ever comes when there is a conflict about your capitation payment, you are at a significant disadvantage.

Referencing Key Documents without Providing a Copy

It is relatively common in managed care contracts to reference key documents in the contract without providing physicians with a copy of the document. The sample definition above references a "Health Services Agreement" that you need to have and review before you sign a contract. Other documents often referenced in contracts include the Quality Improvement Plan, the Utilization Management Plan, the Master Group Contract, and Grievance Procedures. In most instances, you are required to follow the policies and procedures contained in these documents, so you surely need to know what they contain prior to signing a contract.

Covered Services Are Not Clearly Spelled Out

As in the example above, covered services are not always clear. It is imperative that covered services be defined by the CPT code. Later, when there's a dispute about what's covered and what's not, you have all the covered codes at your fingertips. Also, it is important to know the managed care plan's limitations and exclusions. In a capitated system, you certainly don't want to be providing noncovered services as part of your capitation rate. Often, you can provide these services on a fee-for-service basis.

Overcommitment of Provider

Often the managed care plan requires you to commit to providing medical services beyond your current practice capabilities. These may include extending your hours of operation, expanding your on-call system, referring patients to a whole new network of participating specialists and hospitals, handling out-of-area coverage for your patients who are traveling or away at school, scheduling appointments within so many days, and providing data reports to the managed care plan. Before you sign, understand the implications on your practice and make sure you can meet these requirements.

Bad Risk Arrangements

Some managed care plans create risk arrangements that give you financial responsibility but not the authority to control costs. For example, you're at financial risk for inpatient care, but you have no say over who gets admitted, how they get admitted, or the criteria for admission. Other situations can also create problems. You may be at risk for diagnostic tests, but a specialist to whom you made a referral may order a series of expensive tests about which you know nothing. If you are at risk, more often than not, you are completely dependent upon the managed care plan's Utilization Management (UM) department to authorize medically appropriate care. Some UM teams are great, and, unfortunately, some are not. You need to know who pays—the managed care plan or you. If you discover that you pay (usually out of your risk pool), you should at least be able to review pending claims before payment.

No Minimum Enrollment

Insurance is based on the "law of large numbers"—that is, spread your risk of a predicted claim over a large enough population, all of whom are paying you a premium, and you'll make money. As a provider and now as an "insurer" under capitation, you need a large enough member base over which to spread your risk. Many single specialty deals will pay attractive fee-for-service rates up to 2,000 members, after which capitation kicks in. This ensures you more protection than going capitation on the first member.

Exclusivity Requirement

Some managed care plans are requiring exclusivity to get in. They expect you to sign only with them, either because of some past relationships or possible equity positions with them. In such a dynamic and evolving managed care arena where the players buy and sell each other frequently, it is a dangerous strategy to link up with an exclusive deal. Always try to get exclusivity; be extremely careful giving it.

One-Sided Indemnification

Most managed care plans have an indemnification section in their contract. This "indemnifies" or "holds harmless" the other party of the contract in the event of a lawsuit. Watch for indemnification that is one-sided; they require you to indemnify them, but are unwilling to reciprocate. This tells you a lot about the people you'll be working with. Run the language past your attorney and your professional liability carrier before signing.

Poor Termination Provisions

Obviously, if you determine you've entered into a bad deal and you're getting clobbered, you want out—fast. The managed care company, on the other hand, has to find another provider (no easy task if you're getting clobbered) and make arrangements to transfer patients, etc., so they want as much time as they can get to make a smooth transition. The better contracts let you out in 30 days, no questions asked. The worst make you stay in for 180 days without cause and 90 days with cause. Negotiate what works for you. Also, many contracts "automatically renew" on the anniversary date. Avoid this language, if possible. Most contracts that automatically renew are simply filed away and not managed aggressively. The managed care plans don't want to be out there renegotiating every year, but it is in your best interest to revisit the contract at least annually in order to make changes as necessary, including reimbursement changes.

No Detailed Data Reports

Very few managed care plans will spell out and promise you the kind of data reports you need to monitor your risk in a capitated plan. You need detailed data reports to know what's going on with your costs and quality. For example, you need member eligibility reports on the first of the month, member list by age, sex, and plan by the tenth of the month, utilization reports showing all at-risk services with pmpm rates by the fifth of the following month, provider profile reports (specialists and hospitals) by the tenth of the following month, and detailed financial reports showing profits and losses in aggregate, and pmpm by the fifth of the following month.

In summary, risk is not just measured in financial terms. Nonfinancial contract provisions can place you at great risk, and you need to find the hidden risks in each contract you plan to sign.

SUGGESTED READINGS

Beware these common traps when negotiating your next capitation agreement. 1998. *Capitation Management Report* 5, No. 2: 21–23.

Does your capitation contract include these 'Top 12' clauses? 1999. *Capitation Management Report* 6, No. 3: 37–40.

Day 13: Key Assumptions about Your Managed Care Reality

Clifford R. Frank, MHSA

Planning horizons in health care have shrunk from five years to five months. The accelerating pace of change makes orchestrating carefully developed plans into well-executed performance difficult. Most provider groups and organizations are simply staggering from one market calamity to the next. But how individuals and organizations view these changes deeply depends upon their assumptions about how managed care affects markets and about how markets affect managed care.

INPATIENT UTILIZATION IS DECLINING

Use of inpatient hospital services is declining across the nation. This decline is not just the result of a compression of inpatient length of stay, but also is the result of declining admission rates for services that can be performed on an outpatient basis that used to require an inpatient stay. This trend will continue as major procedures move toward alternate site care (such as outpatient hip replacements), alternate procedures performed in lieu of surgery (cardiac stints and minimally invasive surgery), and the need for hospitalization to treat particular diseases is eliminated in many cases (outpatient chemotherapy).

HOSPITAL OUTPATIENT UTILIZATION WILL DECLINE

We used to think that the shift from inpatient to outpatient was about all that was happening. In more advanced managed care markets, hospital outpatient volume also drops as surgical and diagnostic procedures move to physician offices or other low-cost settings. If institutions are anticipating simply transferring the revenue stream from inpatient to outpatient, they may be surprised at the shortfall.

IF SPECIALISTS ARE CAPITATED, SO IS THEIR HOSPITAL— EVEN IF IT'S NOT

We used to think that managing managed care meant getting our specialists on the provider panels of managed care plans. Physicians have done that and more. As physician specialists obtain capitated contracts, their use of procedure-driven care and their use of major diagnostic testing declines substantially. The collateral result is that hospitals that see their physicians obtain capitated contracts for specialty services that used to be provided on a fee-for-service basis will find hospital volumes and revenues in significant decline as the capitation takes hold.

IF SPECIALISTS ARE CAPITATED, THEY MAY BECOME COMPETITORS TO HOSPITALS

As specialists obtain capitated contracts that also include facility costs or specific incentives for facility cost reduction, those capitated specialists will actively seek to either bring selected services such as endoscopy, chemotherapy, nuclear cardiology, and other services into their offices in search of lower costs.

As physicians join together to form groups, they have a ready revenue stream to tap, in the form of moving hospital ancillary services to physician offices.

Physician practice management companies have learned that physicians were not as bad business managers as the practice management companies initially thought. The profit margins from running physician offices more effectively are not enough to sustain Wall Street's appetite for growth in earnings per share. Practice management companies and physicians see the opportunity for selectively unbundling the outpatient service mix at hospitals, and bringing some of those services into their own multispecialty arrangement. Services such as sleep labs, diagnostic centers, physical therapy, outpatient lab, chemotherapy, radiation therapy, and other services are moving out of the hospital to other locales. For hospitals this makes their customers also their competitors and makes evaluating physician behavior more difficult.

THE EMERGENCE OF OPEN-ACCESS HMOs WILL SHAKE MARKETS TO THEIR CORE

Americans love choice. Open-access HMOs, where a patient can go directly to a specialist, sell in the marketplace because employers no longer have to play the heavy in the health care decisions of their employees. Open-access HMOs pay specialists less, but the specialist doesn't have to call the primary care physician for permission to treat the patient. How do narrow network, capitated, or restrictive HMOs compete with the open-access model? They compete in two ways—they broaden access by adding more physicians or adding a point-of-service product option (plan pays 70–80 percent benefit for non-contracting providers), or they lower the price of the restrictive option. If providers are counting on previous exclusive or restrictive network relationships to give them a sustainable market advantage, then open-access products will once again level the playing field.

The emergence of Open-Access HMOs will force hospitals to re-examine their practice acquisitions. If payers move to an open-access model, then what is the care management role of the primary care physician, and how can such physicians direct patients to their employer if patients can bypass them to specialists who may use competing facilities? Hospitals have spent a great deal on primary care acquisition and continue to fund operating losses in primary care. As open-access plans hit the market, hospitals will be forced to look at their acquisition and ongoing funding of operational losses in a new light.

MEDICARE HMOs AND OTHER MEDICARE ARRANGEMENTS ARE GOING TO GROW

Medicare is getting out of the risk bearing business. Traditional Medicare operates at about 2,500 inpatient days/1,000 population per year. Take those same 1,000 people and put them in a Medicare HMO and utilization will drop to about 1,400 days/1,000. Put those 1,000 people in a well-run, capitated system and utilization can fall to 750 days/1,000. And Medicare

HMOs are growing—rapidly. Medicare HMOs grow at the rate of 1 percent market share per month for several years once they are introduced to a market. This lesson has not been lost on the government. With Medicare expense reductions key to the balanced budget agreement, the government is implementing several significant measures to push, pull, induce, seduce, and otherwise help seniors join Medicare managed care programs. For hospitals, utilization is going to fall. For physicians, utilization is going to fall. If you are an ancillary provider, utilization is going to fall. If you are a payer, utilization is going to fall. The strategic question is on what side of the equation do you want to be when utilization falls?

SLOW DECISION MAKING WILL INCREASE ORGANIZATIONAL OPPORTUNITY COSTS

Organizations that engage in lengthy discourse and long decision cycles will find themselves outmaneuvered in the marketplace as change continues to accelerate. Most large organizations' governance structures are not accustomed to responding to substantial market shifts in short periods of time. Yet, as payer/provider alignments form, change, fly apart, and reform, opportunities come and go with little time for paralysis.

SUGGESTED READING

Managed Competition on the Ropes. 1998. *Health Market Survey*, 16 November.

Day 14: How Hospital Managed Care Strategies Affect Physicians

Bruce Ardis, MBA

When hospitals display their annual budget, they typically suppress the last three digits to make the budget easier to read. For solo practitioners, these same suppressed digits can be used to report their average daily practice revenue. Just as hospital budgets are "macro," so are their managed care strategies. When hospitals change their strategies, physician practices can be affected like a rowboat in the wake of an ocean liner.

Since a medical practice can easily be swamped by a hospital's strategy, it is important to understand typical hospital assumptions. Physicians need to recognize these business assumptions hospitals operate under so that they can plan their own future.

Practically every hospital action can be explained by one or more of these assumptions. Physicians will not be surprised by a hospital's managed care strategy if they understand the core values of the hospital and its managers.

HOSPITALS ARE CAPITAL-INTENSIVE ENTERPRISES

First, hospitals are capital-intensive enterprises, and it is essential that they feed the beast. Any business that has significant capital investments must generate an acceptable return on those investments.

New investments will only be made if they can generate an acceptable rate of return on that investment of capital. Physicians use the same process, but the difference is that the primary source of capital for a physician's practice is the intellectual capital of the physician and not a piece of equipment.

HOSPITALS DEFINE SUCCESS IN TERMS OF ADMISSIONS

Second, no matter what administrators say, hospitals define success in terms of admissions—occupied bed days and inpatient market share. There is not one administrator in this country that really believes that a successful managed care strategy will empty the hospital. (A successful managed care strategy will empty a competing hospital and fill the managed care hospital.) Until hospitals stop reporting the average daily census, this will remain THE tool of measurement.

HOSPITALS WANT TO CONTROL THEIR DESTINY

Third, hospitals want to control their destiny. This means they want to control admission sources. To achieve this, hospitals want strategies that guarantee inpatient admissions. This is one reason why so many hospitals are trying to buy primary care practices. They want to control the admissions that those practices generate. If it were not for "Fraud and Abuse," hospitals would obligate practices to admission targets when they purchase a practice.

HOSPITALS BUILD STRATEGY AS IF ALL PATIENTS WERE ON MEDICARE

Finally, since Medicare is typically a hospital's largest payer, hospitals build their strategy as if all patients were Medicare patients.

The exceptions to this rule are inner-city hospitals that may evaluate Medicare and Medicaid as equals and hospitals that specialize in obstetrics that consider commercial patients as the most important. Otherwise most community hospitals will look at the payer world as if Medicare defined it. Investment and service decisions will frequently be made based on how they affect Medicare reimbursement.

Today hospital strategies focus most strongly upon return on investment, control of destiny, and maximizing admissions in developing a strategy. Medicare is the 600-pound gorilla that can start or stop any strategy.

Generally, hospitals make money performing procedures and lose money on medical cases. As a result, the return on investment in equipment used for procedures is high.

Therefore, a hospital will pursue a strategy that increases the number of procedures done using the equipment purchased. When a hospital is not reimbursed at charges, then they will prefer case rates with a Managed Care Organization (MCO). Case rate strategies favor physicians who:

- limit the use of ancillary tests
- use standard supply packs
- use lower-cost implants

In addition, case rates will favor physicians who can bring in low-intensity patients with short lengths of stay. Typically a hospital prefers a practice style that creates low inpatient lengths of stay with rapid discharge to either home health or rehab/subacute care. These secondary services are frequently ones that the hospital is not at risk for as a part of the case rate.

HOSPITALS PURSUE TIGHT PARTNERSHIPS WITH MCOs

One reason hospitals pursue tight partnerships with MCOs is to guarantee volume in some way. Hospitals will seek exclusive arrangements whenever possible since that will limit leakage to competitor hospitals. This strategy will favor physicians who are in that HMO. It can significantly disadvantage physicians active with a competing MCO simply because that MCO may choose to transfer activity to a competing hospital.

The acquisition of physician practices by hospitals is a new challenge for you. There is not just the issue of whether or not you should sell your practice. But any partnership strategy between an MCO and a hospital will have an impact on you—whether or not your practice is acquired by a hospital.

Hospitals will negotiate their most favored deals with HMOs that benefit their practice ownership strategy. Hospitals will look for agreements that maximize hospital or system revenue. It is possible that such an arrangement will not maximize practice revenue. This can force practices not owned by the hospital to contract with those same HMOs under terms that may be less favorable to the practice than what other HMOs and MCOs are offering. The hospital will be negotiating from a global viewpoint, while you are negotiating from a practice perspective. The difficulty will occur if the revenue stream favors institutional services.

Physicians are always at risk when hospitals start doing preferential deals with managed care organizations. If the hospital contracts with the MCO preferred by you, then that is usually not a problem unless it changes your relationship with the MCO. But, what if it is not one of your preferred MCOs? What could be the result? A preferred deal in most hospitals' mind will usually be the one that generates the largest profit/surplus to the hospital. But, one reason the hospital can get more is because the physicians get less. (This is why an MCO deal with a preferred organization by the hospital can affect you.) The impact this has on a physician practice is negative unless the MCO can generate enough additional business to make up for the lost income. Additionally, volume is usually a good thing, especially today when most practices are coping with flat or declining growth.

Sometimes it isn't the fee schedule that is at issue, it is other things. Some MCOs just aren't as easy to work with as others. If the hospital aligns itself with a difficult MCO, then your practice will have increased volume from this difficult MCO. In this case the hospital can cause significant operational problems for physicians that can be difficult to overcome. It is difficult to ask the hospital to offset an increase in your costs that this change has created. Even worse, sometimes the increased administrative burden for your practice is a transfer of administrative burden from the hospital.

In some markets, particularly markets dominated by one hospital, physicians can find themselves as the financial fall guy of the hospital–MCO relationship. The hospital may be very successful at negotiating a rewarding contract. If the HMO cannot find other sources of revenue to offset those increased costs, they will be looking for ways to save. Physician fees are vulnerable, as are professional capitation rates. Too many hospitals do not understand that if inpatient prices are too high, the MCO will find outpatient alternatives. These outpatient alternatives may not be as convenient for you or your patients as your present alternatives. High inpatient prices can also encourage the MCO to increase its police activity. When that occurs, it can be more difficult to get procedures approved and can result in a larger number of retroactive denials to your practice.

Solutions to this scenario vary depending upon the circumstances. The first solution is if you are in a specialty being acquired (usually primary care), you should seriously consider the hospital's offer. Hospitals have recently discovered how difficult it is to manage physician practices.

Because of this, you may be able to negotiate a deal that allows you more practice autonomy in exchange for more of your income being based upon productivity and not salary. Salaried physicians have burned hospitals; therefore, you may be able to negotiate more freedom in your practice. The alternative is to go to the hospital and ask it to join you in your MCO negotiations to help you get additional benefits for your practice. This may force the hospital to take income from its pocket, but it may be willing to do so to preserve a long-term relationship.

If you are a specialist in a specialty that the hospital is not acquiring, your best strategy is to go to the hospital and ask for its assistance in improving your position in the contracts. It may be able to negotiate some risk sharing that benefits you. This strategy needs to be used with care.

Hospitals will seriously consider your needs only if you can demonstrate that its actions are affecting your practice. You have to be able to demonstrate that your income and volume decline was caused by the hospital's actions and not by broader market forces that are causing most physicians in your specialty to suffer. As specialty income goes down, it will be increasingly difficult to demonstrate this. It is important for you to show that volume is being lost from switching from one MCO to another MCO and that the income loss is not associated with lower reimbursement per visit.

Unfortunately reimbursement per visit is declining for all payers, and you can expect it to get worse. A hospital is unlikely to protect you from the effects of the marketplace.

While large physician groups have a chance of controlling their destiny when a hospital changes strategy, smaller practices are at a disadvantage. As you plan, it is important to understand the motivations and assumptions that hospital administrators have. Keeping those in mind may make some actions seem less like an evil plot and more like a self-interested, self-preservation strategy for the hospital. Understanding what motivates a hospital will allow you to develop strategies that enable you to be successful. If you react to hospital changes as "evil actions," you can achieve some moral satisfaction. If you react to the changes as understandable business actions, you can achieve financial satisfaction.

SUGGESTED READINGS

Goldsmith, J. 1993. Driving the Nitroglycerin Truck. *Healthcare Forum Journal* 36, No. 2: 36–44, March/April.

Heimoff, S. 1997. The Reasons Why So Many Hospital-Physician Associations Fall Apart. *Strategic Health Care Marketing* 14, No. 1: 1–5.

Levitt, L. 1999. Finding the Trends in Health Care Chaos. *Managed Care*, July.

Morissey, M.A. et al. 1999. The Effects of Managed Care on Physician and Clinical Integration in Hospitals. *MedCare* 37, No. 4: 350–361.

Ziger, A. 1997. They Made the Right Choice When the Money Ran Low. *Managed Care*, September.

Day 15: How Physician Managed Care Strategies Affect Hospitals

Bruce Ardis, MBA

INTRODUCTION

The strategies physicians employ to respond to managed care are complex and not easily categorized. Part of this is because some physicians have conscious strategies, while others are just going along. The other complicating factor is that the appropriate response is dependent upon each physician's specialty and/or the kind of practice he or she is in. Also, group practices face different opportunities and challenges than a solo practitioner.

ORGANIZED OR DISORGANIZED PHYSICIANS?

All of this makes it very difficult for hospitals to develop a physician-sensitive managed care strategy. It is probable that a hospital will be responding to a dozen or so strategies.

There are two rough categories of physician response for hospitals to deal with. The first is the disorganized physician staff consisting of small groups and solo practitioners. In this scenario, the groups are usually single specialty and typically are specialists.

The second category exists when there are one or more large multispecialty group practices. This kind of organized group can usually leverage hospitals and health plans to do their bidding.

Disorganized Physicians, Weak HMO Steering

The key for hospitals for dealing with a disorganized physician community is to identify the strength of managed care, especially HMOs in the community. If the HMOs are focused on member growth and use large networks to attract members, then it is likely that they have weak hospital steering mechanisms.

The strategy to employ with physicians in these circumstances is to make practicing at your hospital easy. As long as the staff (primaries and specialists) are in the networks, the hospital can control its destiny by emphasizing service to the physicians. Make sure that the physicians can get convenient operating room schedules, timely data from lab, and prompt scheduling from radiology, for example. Competing based on service can allow a hospital to yield above average returns on its managed care contracts.

Disorganized Physicians, Strong HMO Steering

In this environment, the HMOs steer patients to the hospitals that they prefer. Physicians feel that they must respond to the pressures of the plan. Generally, price is the issue for the health plan. The physicians may have incentives that encourage them to direct patients to a particular hospital besides the plans' price incentives.

In this circumstance, the hospital needs to work with the HMOs to be a desired provider. Usually this will mean achieving the price and efficiency objectives of the HMO.

If Specialists Don't Participate

If you have a specialty community that has chosen not to participate in managed care, the strategies above will not work. No matter how much your primaries want to admit patients to your hospital, they can't do it without the surgeons and medical specialists who provide the bulk of inpatient care. In this situation, you need to get your specialists immediately into the managed care plans in which your PCPs have significant membership.

In many areas of the country, HMOs are not admitting new specialists. When that happens, you may have to recruit to your staff specialists who are already participating with the managed care plans. Many staff development plans do not allow for expansion of the size of the medical staff, especially for specialists. This can put you in a "no win" situation: You can't get specialists in a network, and you can't get new physicians on your staff. Even when a staff development plan allows you to add specialists, doing so can be a politically dangerous thing to do. It is possible to approach some HMOs and get them to recruit some of your specialists, but they are unlikely to agree to recruit a large number.

Organized Physicians

Large multispecialty group practices are best able to control their future.
For the hospital, this can be the most difficult situation. It is very easy to be in a bidding war with another hospital and become a pure commodity to be bought and sold at the lowest price. Well-run groups with a clear strategic vision are in a stronger position.

COMPETITION WITH HOSPITALS

Physicians, whether they are organized or disorganized, can compete with the hospital for some basic services. They can take these services out of the hospital and into their offices through managed care contracts. Groups have more capital and can do so more easily, but small, single specialty groups can compete just as effectively with the hospital.

Physicians can set up ambulatory surgical suites either in their offices or in a freestanding center. These suites have low costs when compared to those set up by a hospital. The capital cost can be very low when the suite is used for a single specialty. This is particularly true for endoscopy suites.

Physicians can establish these suites and steal the low- and medium-intensity cases from the hospital by competing on price and convenience when contracting for patients with managed care companies. If hospitals are pricing these services to create operating margins, HMOs can and do contract with other facilities to generate pricing pressure on hospital outpatient services.

Examples of other services that are vulnerable in this environment include radiology and physical therapy.

CARVE-OUT BIDDING

HMO network downsizing is encouraging physicians to think differently. It used to be that open-heart surgery was the big case rate procedure. Since only tertiary facilities were doing these case rate carve-outs, it didn't seem a threat to most community hospitals.

Now orthopedists are putting together package rates (including the hospital) for major joint replacement (DRG 209). Since almost every hospital does joint replacement, suddenly many hospitals are vulnerable to this strategy. Physicians control the protocols.

HMOs can easily leverage one hospital against another. This leaves the successful hospital with marginal costs and a minimal, if any, share of the savings generated by good medical management.

SURVIVAL STRATEGIES, CAVEATS

Because there are so many physicians with conflicting interests, there is not one solution. Any managed care strategy will cause some loss of physician loyalty simply because any strategy appears to favor some physicians at the expense of others. Hospitals must communicate to their staff that their goal is to receive as much directed volume as possible. Maximizing volume has the best chance of benefiting all members of the staff.

The response to the large multispecialty group practice is clear to define but can be very difficult to carry out. Working closely with a group should make the hospital an indispensable, long-term partner. The difficulty for the hospital is that the more joint ventures done with such a group, the more the hospital is perceived as having taken sides in the community. The group's competitors will see the hospital as working against their interests. Ultimately they may be right, but it is very difficult for a hospital to turn its back on a large group and survive.

CONCLUSION

Even as this is written, physicians are developing new strategies that will demand fresh solutions. Be ready to change with them. But pursuing these unbundling strategies can trigger a hostile response from hospitals, and physicians need to think through the downstream consequences before embarking on this path.

SUGGESTED READINGS

Goldsmith, J. 1993. Driving the Nitroglycerin Truck. *Healthcare Forum Journal* 36, No. 2: 36–44, March/April.

Heimoff, S. 1997. The Reasons Why So Many Hospital-Physician Associations Fall Apart. *Strategic Health Care Marketing* 14, No. 1: 1–5.

Levitt, L. 1999. Finding the Trends in Health Care Chaos. *Managed Care*, July.

Ziger, A. 1997. They Made the Right Choice When the Money Ran Low. *Managed Care*, September.

Day 16: Using Rate Filings to Your Advantage

Joel Hornberger, MHS

How would you like to be playing cards with a Las Vegas blackjack dealer and know what cards he's holding, which card he's going to deal, and in what order he's going to deal them? Most of us would love to see the other guy's cards—in Vegas or in business. Well, studying managed care rate filings is a lot like looking at a managed care exec's cards. Managed care firms are required to file a gold mine of service and financial data to certain regulatory bodies in your state, usually the State Insurance Department. These data then become public information, and you or anyone else can look at them and, in most cases, copy them. (Managed care firms usually pay thousands of dollars to actuarial companies for these data, and you can get the data for your time and copy expense!) With these data, you will know exactly what the managed care company is assuming its utilization and costs will be, and you will see exactly what it is budgeting for primary care services, specialty services, ER, lab, x-ray, OB, administrative overhead, and profit, as well as a wealth of other health services. When the managed care negotiator comes knocking on your hospital or physician practice door with a capitation contract in hand, you will already know the numbers he or she is holding.

ACCESSING RATE FILINGS

The first thing you have to do is get the data. This is usually fairly simple. Find out who regulates managed care firms in your state, call them, and tell them you want to make an appointment to review some rate filings. Ask them at that time to explain their copying procedures, fees, and preferred method of payment (cash or check). Almost always, you will have to go physically to their office. When you show up, someone will take you to the rate filings area. You may have to sign in and out, and sometimes sign out and sign back in the actual rate filings.

READING RATE FILINGS

Summary and Narrative Parts of the Rate Filing

Rate filings look complicated and difficult to read, but once you know what you're looking for, they're pretty easy to read. First, the rate filings will be organized alphabetically by company name. If you are researching a particular company, you simply pull that company's rate filing. Second, the rate filing will be organized by date of submission. Usually, the first time a company files in the state, there is a long, detailed rate filing with a gold mine of data. Thereafter, they can often file amendments to the original document. Each rate filing will be dated. Make sure you get the original document plus all the amendments so you can identify price and/or utilization trends and assumptions. Finally, they may be organized by plan or product (e.g., a $5 copayment plan, a $10 copayment plan, etc.). Make sure you know which plan or product you're looking at.

Next, you will see summary information (usually in narrative form) and detailed tables. You'll be tempted to go right to the detailed tables, but don't overlook the narrative part of the document. Often it describes marketing strategies, enrollment projections, overall utilization or price assumptions, inflationary assumptions, reinsurance arrangements, and any special capitation carve-outs the managed care firm has already negotiated (e.g., behavioral health, cardiology, orthopedic, etc.). After you have reviewed the summary information and narrative, you will want to dive into the detailed tables.

Rate Filing Detailed Tables

Table II–3 shows you what a typical rate filing table might look like. Don't panic if your table looks slightly different than this one. The formats are often different, but the content is pretty much the same.

Table II–3 Hospital Inpatient Services: Sample Rate Filing Tables

SERVICES	UTIL/K	GROSS CHARGE	GROSS PMPM	COPAY OFFSET	NET PMPM
Medical Days	123 days/k	$ 1,486.55	$ 15.23	$0	$ 15.23
Surgical Days	109 days/k	$ 1,558.48	$ 14.16	$0	$ 14.16
Psych Days	————	————	$ 2.25	————	$ 2.25
Maternity Days	39 days/k	$ 1,456.60	$ 4.73	$0	$ 4.73
TOTAL	321 days	————	$ 51.24	————	$ 51.24

Across the top of the rate filing, you will see a number of column headings. On the far left, you will see "Services." This comes from an actuary looking at the benefit plan and determining what medical benefits are covered or excluded. If there are numbers filled in across the rows, it is a covered benefit; if there are zeros filled in across the rows, it is an excluded service.

The next column usually is "Utilization/K" or "Frequency." This is an actuarial projection of how many services will be used by 1,000 covered lives under the plan per year. Actuaries use databases, claims history, product design, and population covered to project utilization of services. The next column is an actuarial estimate of how much the HMO expects to pay for a unit of service (e.g., per day or per visit or per procedure, etc.). This is often based on geographic health care costs, but can also be based on deals the HMO has already negotiated or expects to negotiate.

The next column is usually labeled "Gross PMPM" or "PMPM." It is developed by taking the "Utilization/K" column times the "Gross Charge" column and dividing by 12,000. The reason they divide by 12,000 is because the utilization figure is expressed as per 1,000 members per year, and they want to get it down to per member per month. Thus, you have to divide by 1,000 to get "per member" and by 12 to get "per month."

The next column is often labeled "Copay." This comes from the benefit plan design and is the amount the patient pays at the time he or she receives a particular service. Often, an HMO will require the patient to pay $10 for an office visit or $100 for outpatient surgery.

The last column shows the "Net PMPM." This is the Gross PMPM minus any copayments expected from the patient. To get the Copayment PMPM, you simply take the Utilization/K or Frequency times the Copayment amount shown and divide by 12,000. You then subtract the Copayment PMPM from the Gross PMPM to get "Net PMPM."

In Table II–3, the HMO is projecting 123 days/k for medical days, with an average per diem of $1,486.55. Multiplying these two numbers and dividing by 12,000 gives you $15.23 per member per month. There is no copayment by the patient at the time of service, so the net PMPM is also $15.23. Surgical days are similarly structured.

Looking at Psych services from Table II–3, you see they do not have any utilization or charge information. Why not? Because the HMO has subcontracted Psych to a Behavioral Health company for $2.25. Since this is fixed, it is "plugged" into the rate filing. Increasingly, MCOs are shifting risk to providers under capitation contracts, so you might see similar

Table II–4 Physician Services

SERVICES	UTIL/K	GROSS CHARGE	GROSS PMPM	COPAY OFFSET	NET PMPM
Inpatient Surgery	54 Procs	$ 1,887.96	$ 8.50	$ 0	$ 8.50
Outpatient Surgery	400 Procs	$ 384.92	$ 12.83	$ 100.00	$ 9.50
Inpatient Visits	295 Visits	$ 98.80	$ 2.43	$ 0	$ 2.43
Vision, Hearing, Speech	0	0	0	0	0
Chiropractic Services	168 Visits	$ 46.29	$ .65	$ 10.00	$ .51
Office Visits	2,146.5 Visits	$ 52.00	$ 9.30	$ 10.00	$ 7.51

"plugs" for cardiology, orthopedic, etc. This is great information if you are trying to get the contract away from an existing provider, since you can see exactly what the current fee is.

Physician services follow the same pattern as above, except you will usually see more copayments for physician services (see Table II–4). The "Outpatient Surgery" benefit for this MCO must require the patient to pay a $100 copayment at the time of service. You can see that the actuaries are projecting 400 outpatient surgeries per 1,000 members per year at an average charge of $384.92. Multiplying these two numbers together and dividing by 12,000 gives you the $12.83 gross pmpm. Taking the 400 surgeries times the $100 copayment, and dividing by 12,000 gives you $3.33 pmpm, which is subtracted from the $12.83 to give you $9.50. Similar math follows for physician Office Visits and Chiropractic Visits, since they have a $10 copayment. If you're a chiropractor and the MCO comes to you with a capitation deal of $.30 pmpm, it's nice to know that they're really budgeting $.51 pmpm!

Also, note that it appears Vision, Hearing, and Speech are excluded benefits since the MCO is assuming no utilization. These services may be excluded, but the MCO may be assuming that these services are included in basic physician office visits. Check the contract to see.

Data will help you make more informed decisions. Armed with Rate Filing data, you're in a much better position to know which services are covered and which ones are not, projected utilization, projected costs, benefit plan copayments, and resulting capitation rates. All these data will help you make more informed decisions about your capitation contracting and will give you a peek at the other guy's cards.

Day 17: TennCare Managed Medicaid

Joel Hornberger, MHS

On New Year's Day, 1994, Tennessee health care providers woke up to a new era of health care delivery. As bowl games were fought on televisions all over the U.S., Tennessee health care providers were about to be crushed by a politically driven health care system known as TennCare. A new managed Medicaid program, TennCare would become for many providers a continuous hangover that New Year's Day, changing forever the way in which they cared for people. Unprepared providers from the Great Smoky Mountains to Music Row to the great porticos of Graceland felt shock waves. The message was clear early on—adapt to managed care or die.

This article will not debate the pros and cons of TennCare, as there are many of each, but instead will focus on helping providers in other Medicaid waiver states learn important lessons from the TennCare experience and apply them to their practices and facilities.

LESSON 1—YOU MUST DEVELOP NEW POLITICAL SKILLS AND ALLIANCES

Managed Medicaid is driven by politics and money, pure and simple. It's about state governors, state legislators, state bureaucrats, state committees, and federal bureaucrats all trying to save public monies—savings coming, for the most part, out of the providers' pockets. The political rhetoric is about increasing coverage for the poor, improving access to needed health care services, and enhancing quality of care; but the bottom line is the control or reduction of benefit costs.

Providers must develop strong political skills and use them aggressively. You must get involved in the political arena. You must lobby. You must form PACs and write checks to them. Don't depend on your Association to carry the ball; you need to get in the game. You can't afford to fail to influence the political creation of new health care delivery systems in your state.

You can't depend on your professional Associations alone. The Tennessee Medical Association and the Tennessee Hospital Association, both powerful and well-funded organizations, were unable to make the kinds of changes to TennCare they wanted, even with the threat or reality of lawsuits and intense lobbying.

TennCare was created literally overnight, with many providers and provider Associations caught off-guard. In off-the-record talks with state officials, it became clear that the sudden screeching implementation of the program was actually planned and purposeful, designed as a "surprise air strike" on the Medicaid system before providers could mount any meaningful resistance. Providers are out of business today because they failed to recognize the political threats years before TennCare became a reality.

LESSON 2—YOU MUST DEVELOP STRONG CONTRACT NEGOTIATION SKILLS

HCFA's main concern, in their approval of any state Medicaid waiver, is access to an adequate number of primary care and specialty providers. The last thing they want are newspaper stories about poor children dying or suffering because they can't find a provider who will take Medicaid.

Tennessee's providers, unaccustomed for the most part to capitation and managed care, were unenthusiastic about signing early TennCare contracts. If they didn't sign, the State could not come close to proving to HCFA that TennCare had an adequate network of providers. So the Blues came to the State's rescue with a controversial and highly criticized "cram down" policy. The "cram down" required that a provider must participate in TennCare if they participate in the Blues' huge commercial PPO, which served the lucrative state employees and private business markets. By leveraging their tremendous market share power, the Blues had the providers right where they wanted them. Large numbers of physicians dropped out of the commercial products, but nearly all came back months later when their anger and income had diminished.

Contracting lessons? First, make sure your current contracts do not have a provision whereby they become invalid if you refuse to participate in other less desirable company "products." You need the flexibility to analyze each deal (capitation rate, fee schedule, etc.) presented to you and not be forced to take a bad deal just so you can continue with the managed care company. Pull out your current contracts and see if you're required to participate in any of the company products. See what happens if you refuse the deal that's offered. Also, see if the MCO can force one-sided contract amendments. Focus on your big contracts (like your Blues' deal) because that's where you're most vulnerable to a shift of your patients. If you find contracts with a potential "cram down," begin negotiating!

Second, you must understand that state Medicaid programs moving to managed care are in the business of shifting risk to YOU. Consequently, you must understand risk. You must be able to analyze whether the deal is terrible or not, how much risk you are willing and able to accept, the kind of risk being transferred to other providers in the system and its impact on you, and how much it's going to cost you to implement risk management strategies.

LESSON 3—DEVELOP YOUR CAPITATION MANAGEMENT SKILLS

TennCare has seen several providers become big winners. These managed care winners have developed risk management skills designed to maximize their capitation payments while providing quality care. They understand the new realities of managed care budgeting by per member per month. They know utilization rates. They know their costs (absolutely critical in TennCare and any managed care system!). They have or are developing solid management information systems that give them accurate, timely reports. They are willing to accept controllable risk because they've developed internal utilization management, quality assurance programs, and other risk management infrastructure.

Providers interested in learning lessons from TennCare must develop and implement an organizational infrastructure that manages financial risk while providing quality health care. Your MIS must be flexible, powerful, and managed care ready. Some systems need to be able to pay claims, perform utilization authorizations, and track customer services inquiries depending on the provider's risk arrangements. Your staff must be trained and must understand the different (and opposing) revenue maximization strategies in transitioning from a fee-for-service system to a capitated system.

LESSON 4—BEWARE OF THE ATTORNEY GENERAL AND THE ANTITRUST SQUAD

When providers see familiar environments changing and feel the heat of increased risk, they tend to join forces, reasoning that bigger is better. Often it is, but joining forces must be done carefully in order to avoid antitrust exposure.

TennCare saw several serious antitrust investigations of competing providers allegedly collaborating with one another, boycotting managed care organizations, fixing prices, or excluding other competitors. The Tennessee Attorney General and the Tennessee Bureau of Investigation swooped into numerous providers' offices, most notably behavioral health providers, and subpoenaed truckloads of original documents.

Clearly, antitrust is serious, complicated, and costly. Attorney generals aggressively prosecute "white collar" crime, especially when highly paid doctors and hospital administrators are involved. HCFA and other federal agencies are pursuing an aggressive campaign to fight white-collar crime in health care, and the recent Columbia investigations are only the tip of the iceberg. You must have excellent legal advice and a second opinion from an experienced antitrust attorney if you are talking with other providers about anything other than the weather!

LESSON 5—DEVELOP THE CAPABILITY OF EXCEEDING ESTABLISHED PERFORMANCE CRITERIA

TennCare bureaucrats have decided to make "quality" and "access" tangible through numerous performance measures. Essentially, they have developed a provider "report card" and are measuring performance in areas of appointment scheduling, waiting room times, telephone answering time, on-call arrangements, etc. One contract with a managed care organization had over 200 performance measures (developed with little or no provider input).

You should get copies of performance measures from TennCare, other states, HCFA, and managed care organizations to see what your "report card" will most likely look like, and then develop the internal capabilities to score high. The National Committee on Quality Assurance (NCQA) audit criteria provides excellent insight into what MCOs are facing by accrediting bodies. Provider "profiling" is increasingly important to managed care companies as they attempt to change practice patterns of "outliers" or "poor quality" providers.

LESSON 6—PLAN!

Most health care providers were unprepared for TennCare because they failed to plan for eventual managed care change. You must conduct good, solid strategic planning if you are going to thrive in a managed Medicaid world. This planning needs to take a cold, hard look at your organization's strengths and weaknesses. It needs to identify opportunities and threats in your market.

Your planning must result in clear, well-communicated goals; concise, measurable objectives; and specific action steps designed to accomplish your goals and objectives. You need detailed plans for each of the following areas: finances, operations, facilities, computer and MIS, utilization management, quality assurance, strategic alliances, lobbying, managed care contracting, risk assumption, and risk management.

It is a good idea to take your strategic plan and fold it into a business plan. This allows you, and potential investors, to see multiyear balance sheets, income statements, cash flow statements, and return on investment.

The old adage is true: "Most people don't plan to fail, they fail to plan." Start planning today. If you wait to plan, the sweeping managed care changes will overtake you so suddenly that you will be constantly reacting to them rather than shaping them.

LESSON 7—UNDERSTAND AND USE PROVIDER GRIEVANCE PROCEDURES

Grievance procedures are a big deal with HCFA and state bureaucrats. All states (and contracted MCOs) undertaking managed Medicaid "reform" are required to have detailed grievance procedures in place and communicated to consumers and providers. Under TennCare, consumers have filed grievances, but providers have been reluctant to do so.

Not using the grievance procedures is a huge mistake for providers. The grievance procedures state specific time frames for resolving the problem, and that's what providers need when no one responds to their concerns. If all providers filed grievances when they have a legitimate concern or problem, the MCOs would not be able to handle the volume!

Under TennCare, the administrative problems were many: Some MCOs weren't paying claims correctly or at all, eligibility lists weren't being distributed, MCO monitoring by the State was not occurring as required, MCO telephone systems weren't working or were too busy to get through, and the list goes on. Providers "whined" (according to one state senator), but for the most part did not file grievances. You must not let the MCOs or their subcontractors dismiss your concerns by patting your head and sending you on your way, you must file grievances tactfully and properly, using the tool they gave you, in order to raise problems to the level where they can be fixed. You owe it to yourself and to your patients.

LESSON 8—GET THE BEST COMPUTER AND MIS SYSTEM MONEY CAN BUY

Although mentioned briefly above, this lesson is so important it deserves more discussion. Managed care is about data—data that tell you utilization rates, costs, quality, outcomes, patient satisfaction, etc. Your computer system must be able to handle capitation accounting, utilization management tracking and authorizations, referral tracking and authorizations, claims payment if you're subcontracting care to another entity that you have to pay, provider profiling, provider compensation (including contact capitation methodologies), patient demographics, online eligibility verification, and Internet and/or intranet capabilities, to name a few.

Many providers under TennCare (or any managed care system for that matter) have no idea if their pmpm costs are exceeding their pmpm revenues. Their computer systems simply will not allow them to get the data. This is a lot like General Motors knowing the price of a car on the dealer's lot, but not having any idea how much it cost them to make it and get it there. If their costs exceed their price, they're not going to be around long. And so it is with providers—your computer system must allow you to know your pmpm costs by type of service, by provider, by month compared to your pmpm revenues.

Frankly, most providers' computer systems can't cut it. One provider under TennCare lost over $300,000 because it couldn't verify a particular category of patient! It is reasonable to estimate that providers lost millions of dollars in TennCare because their computer systems couldn't handle the data demands.

LESSON 9—KNOW HOW TO CALCULATE CAPITATION RATES

Many providers in TennCare, even years after being paid by capitation, still don't know how to calculate capitation rates. There is a resistance by many providers to understand what is a very simple mathematical formula. Its key factors are services, utilization rates, and costs.

Understanding how capitation calculations work is vitally important because it is the way an MCO budgets for health care services. For example, primary care services may be budgeted at 2,000 visits per 1,000 members (per year) at an assumed cost of $30 per visit. Multiplying these two numbers and dividing by 12,000 (to get per member per month), you have a "budget" of $5.00 pmpm (2,000 x 30 ÷ 12,000). This is done for the whole mix of medical services provided under the Medicaid or TennCare benefit package.

By understanding this simple calculation, you can see the important implications for data, MIS systems, utilization management, cost accounting by pmpm, operations, provider profiling, etc. It puts the lessons above into an understandable managed care context.

LESSON 10—CHANGE

Last, but not least, TennCare taught providers they must change. Those that refused to change are no longer in business. Those organizations that were able to adapt, to recognize the new realities of health care delivery, and change to take advantage of them, have survived.

The greatest changes TennCare providers experienced have been:

- a radical new shifting of financial risk away from the state and MCO to providers

- a new competitive order whereby market share and "covered lives is the name of the game"
- a new emphasis on data and reporting to MCOs and the state
- a need to manage the risk being shifted to them
- a reallocation of scarce medical resources away from the inpatient setting to the outpatient and office setting
- health care delivery being organized by the state via political and economic pressures.

Day 18: Managed Care Resource Guide

Clifford R. Frank, MHSA

The managed care information options available to each of us are expanding rapidly, but knowing which are worthwhile and which are a waste of time is difficult. The following lists (Exhibits II–1 through II–7) will provide you with some time-tested high-quality information sources that are worthy of your consideration. These lists, while comprehensive in scope, are not wholly complete as new publications, associations, websites, and other information sources continually develop. This set of information sources provides timely, reliable, comprehensive, and detailed information that will be useful to the day-to-day managed care professional. Some of these publications overlap in several areas so that selecting carefully can save you money.

SUGGESTED READINGS

Chang, C.F. et al. 1998. Tennessee's Failed Managed Care Program for Mental Health and Substance Abuse Services. *The Journal of the American Medical Association* 279, No. 11: 864–869.

Wade, P. 1998. No New Money for TennCare Despite Recommendations, State Officials Say. *The Commercial Appeal*, 19 March.

Wade, P. 1998. State Investigating if TennCare Tried To Have Reports Doctored. *The Commercial Appeal*, 31 December.

1998. Tennessee CMHC lawsuit could alter troubled managed care program. *Mental Health Weekly* 8, No. 23

Exhibit II–1 Managed Care—General Industry Information Sources

Name of Publication	Description	Contact Information
The Advisory Board Company	This subscription research organization provides excellent topical research findings and presentations on managed care and other important areas. The Advisory Board publications are only available to member organizations and membership is restricted to certain types of health care organizations.	The Watergate 600 New Hampshire Avenue N.W. Washington, DC 20037 202/672-5600 202/672-5700 (fax)
Health Affairs	This journal, published quarterly, often has some of the most thoughtful articles from a variety of perspectives about managed care issues. The journal publishes articles from some of the more notable health economists and health system leaders while also providing commentary on socio-political trends of our day.	Health Affairs P.O. Box 148 Congers, NY 10920 800/765-7514 914/267-3479 (fax)
The Interstudy Competitive Edge	Quarterly reports on HMO enrollment by product type, plan age and many other useful variables. Also includes basic utilization rates for plans.	Interstudy Publications P.O. Box 4366 St. Paul, MN 55104 612/ 858-9291 612/854-5698 (fax)
Managed Care Digest Series	This series of reports is published annually on medical groups, integrated health care systems, and HMO/PPO organizations. Data on group size, administrative costs, utilization rates, PMPM expenditures, profit margins, and other valuable information is included.	Hoechst Marion Roussel P.O. Box 9627 Kansas City, MO 64134 800/552-3656 816/966-3860 (fax)
Pulse	This newsletter provides market, financial, and operating statistics for HMOs on a monthly basis. Financial ratios, operating results, and comparative information are published along with topical news on industry segments.	Sherlock Company P.O. Box 413 Gwynedd, PA 19436 215/628-2289 215/542-0690 (fax) E-mail: sherlock@sherlockco.com Website: www.sherlockco.com
Russ Coile's Health Trends	This monthly newsletter provides insights into changes in the health care field, including managed care, by looking at macro societal and economic trends to figure out how those play out in health care markets.	Aspen Publishers, Inc. 7201 McKinney Circle Frederick, MD 21704 301/698-7100 301/695-7931 (fax)

Exhibit II–2 Managed Care—General News Services

Name of Publication	Description	Contact Information
Health Market Survey	Excellent concise reports on specific activities of plans, providers, and the government from a pro-HMO editorial viewpoint.	Interpro Publications Inc. P.O. Box 9902, Friendship Station Washington, DC 20016 202/362-5408 202/362-0984 (fax)
Healthcare Practice Management News	Provides business intelligence on acquisitions, alliances, technology, and other developments.	Business Information Services, Inc. 12811 North Point Lane Laurel, MD 20708 800/559-8550 301/604-5126 (fax)
Managed Care Outlook	Coverage of national managed care issues with limited coverage of local/regional issues.	Aspen Publishers, Inc. 200 Orchard Ridge Drive #200 Gaithersburg, MD 20878 301/417-7500
Managed Care Reporter	Broad treatment of managed care issues.	Bureau of National Affairs 9435 Keywest Avenue Rockville, MD 20850 800/372-1033 800/253-0332 (fax)
Managed Care Week	Good political reporting and reporting of major managed care developments.	Atlantic Information Services, Inc. 1100 17th Street N.W., Suite 300 Washington, DC 20036 202/775-9008 202/331-9542 (fax)
Managed Healthcare News	Trade publication that covers selected managed care topics and current news developments.	Quadrant HealthCom Inc. 26 Main Street Chatham, NJ 07928 973/701-8900 973/701-8892 (fax) www.managedhealthcarenews.com
Managed Healthcare Market Report	Newsletter containing competitive analysis for providers and purchasers of managed care.	Corporate Research Group Inc. 524 North Avenue, Suite 302 New Rochelle, NY 10801 914/235-6000 914/235-6002 (fax) E-mail: corpsrch@aol.com

Exhibit II–3 Managed Care—Practical Information

Name of Publication	Description	Contact Information
Capitation Abstracts & Analysis	A monthly digest and critique of capitation literature.	Advisory Publications 15 E. Ridge Pike, Suite 510 Conshohocken, PA 19428-2124 888/941-4488 610/941-4499 (fax) E-mail: fordocs@aol.com
Capitation Management Report	This monthly publication provides useful comparisons, details on capitation, and cost-cutting arrangements under managed care.	National Health Information, LLC 1123 Zonolite Road, Suite 24 Atlanta, GA 30306-2016 800/597-6300 770/998-2434 (fax) E-mail: nhi@nhionline.net Website: www.nhionline.net
Capitation Rates and Data	This publication provides information on risk contracting through real-world examples. Illustrative data are routinely presented and interesting success stories are reported. Some of the data presented are quirky, so use carefully.	National Health Information, LLC P.O. Box 670505 Marietta, GA 30066 800/597-6300 770/998-2434 (fax) E-mail: nhinfo@aol.com
Data Strategies & Benchmarks	A monthly advisory for health care executives.	National Health Information, LLC 1123 Zonolite Road, Suite 24 Atlanta, GA 30306-2016 800/597-6300 770/998-2434 (fax) E-mail: nhi@nhionline.net Website: www.nhionline.net
Eli Medicare Risk	This bimonthly publication is designed to provide accurate and authoritative information regarding news, trends, and strategies for managed Medicare.	Eli Research 2327 Englert Drive, Suite 202 Durham, NC 27713 800/874-9180 919/544-3147 (fax) E-mail: geyerl@eliresearch.com
Managed Care Contract Negotiator	A monthly publication that provides actual contract language, negotiating techniques, and working tools helpful in dealing with managed care plans.	Brownstone Publishers, Inc. 149 Fifth Avenue New York, NY 10010-6801 800/643-8095 212/473-8786 (fax) E-mail: lawpub@aol.com
Physician Capitation Report	This monthly newsletter provides news, analysis, and resources for capitated physicians. It provides in-depth reporting into sophisticated managed care issues. The newsletter is very useful to managed care managers who have gotten beyond their first risk contract and want to enhance their understanding of the subtleties of risk contracting. The reference section at the end of each article with contact information for persons quoted in the article is particularly helpful.	Ingenix Publishing (formerly St. Anthony Publishing, Inc.) 11410 Isaac Newton Square Reston, VA 20190 800/632-0123 703/707-5700 (fax)
Physician's Managed Care Report	This monthly newsletter provides a sampling of managed care activity around the country without overwhelming the reader with specifics. The newsletter also has a contact list for persons referenced in each issue.	American Health Consultants 3525 Piedmont Road, N.E. Building 6, Suite 400 Atlanta, GA 30305 800/688-2421 800/284-3291 (fax) E-mail: custserv@ahcpub.com
Public Sector Contracting Report	This is an excellent monthly newsletter that describes with great specificity the challenges and opportunities of managed care today. Most of its content is on managed Medicare and Medicaid, but other topics are covered. Practical suggestions, interesting data, and important lessons learned are included in most every issue.	National Health Information, LLC 4343 Shallowford Road Building B, Suite 8B Marietta, GA 30062 800/597-6300 770/998-2434 (fax) E-mail: nhi@nhionline.net Website: www.nhionline.net

Exhibit II–4 Managed Care—Strategy Newsletters

Name of Publication	Description	Contact Information
Health Plan Business (formerly Managed Care Law Outlook)	This monthly newsletter has gone beyond reporting the latest legal developments and has moved to helping readers think through the implications of those cases.	Aspen Publishers, Inc. 200 Orchard Ridge Drive #200 Gaithersburg, MD 20878 301/417-7500
Health System Leader	This monthly newsletter uses a very thoughtful case-study approach to describe various health systems' strategies and implementation challenges. The newsletter often has material suitable as educational information to others in your organization.	Aspen Publishers, Inc. 200 Orchard Ridge Drive #200 Gaithersburg, MD 20878 301/417-7500
Integrated Healthcare Report	This monthly newsletter provides excellent market-by-market analysis of the maneuverings, machinations, and angst felt by providers, payers, and employers as managed care causes market changes. This newsletter is definitely one to pass around the office.	Integrated Healthcare P.O. Box 839 Lake Arrowhead, CA 92352-0839 909/336-1586 909/336-1567 (fax) Website: www.ihr-ihs.com
Medical Network Strategy Report	This monthly newsletter is designed to help hospital executives develop physician linkage strategies, with managed care as a part of those strategies.	Core Healthcare Resources P.O. Box 40959 Santa Barbara, CA 93140-0959 805/564-2177 805/564-2146 (fax)

Exhibit II–5 Practice Management Company Information

Name of Publication	Description	Contact Information
Healthcare Practice Management News	This monthly publication provides news, analysis, and commentary about practice management companies and their strategies, targets, and vulnerabilities.	Business Information Services, Inc. 12811 North Point Lane Laurel, MD 20708 301/604-4001 301/604-5126 (fax)
Inside PPMCs	This biweekly newsletter provides up-to-date information on PPMC acquisitions, mergers, and contracts. Contact names and phone numbers are also included.	Atlantic Information Services, Inc. 1100 17th Street, N.W., Suite 300 Washington, DC 20036 800/521-4323 202/331-9542 (fax)
PPMC	This monthly newsletter does for practice management companies what *Pulse* does for HMOs. Fascinating information in a wildly changing industry.	Sherlock Company P.O. Box 413 Gwynedd, PA 19436 215/628-2289 215/542-0690 (fax) E-mail: sherlock@sherlockco.com
Physician Practice Management Report	News from the practice management front lines twice monthly.	Corporate Research Group Inc. 524 North Avenue, Suite 302 New Rochelle, NY 10801 914/235-6000 914/235-6002 (fax) E-mail: corpsrch@aol.com

Exhibit II–6 Associations

Name of Association	Description	Contact Information
The Alliance for Healthcare Strategy and Marketing	The Alliance has broadened its focus to include a great deal of managed care information. Its forward-looking meetings are always put together well and filled with new ideas.	11 S. LaSalle Street, Suite 2300 Chicago, IL 60603 312/704-9700 312/704-9709 (fax)
American Association of Health Plans	This association represents HMOs and PPOs. Its annual meeting is usually well attended and its policy forum is usually the largest winter meeting of the industry.	1129 20th Street, N.W., Suite 600 Washington, DC 20036-3403 202/778-3200 202/331-7487 (fax)
Healthcare Financial Management Association	This association is comprised of financial managers from the health care industry and offers reliably good continuing education programs in managed care.	2 Westbrook Corporate Center Suite 700 Westchester, IL 60153 800/252-4362 708/531-0032 (fax)
The IPA Association of America	This association provides services that will assist in improving the overall operations of IPAs nationwide. To help serve the varying educational needs of its members, TIPAAA holds an annual national meeting.	333 Hegenberger Road, Suite 305 Oakland, CA 94621 510/569-6561 510/569-2753 (fax) E-mail: TIPAAA@aol.com
National Association of Integrated Health Organizations	This association is comprised of group practices, medical centers, health systems, and other providers. It holds three major national conferences and publish a monthly newsletter called *PSO-IHO Report*.	2217 Princess Anne Street Suite 201-1 Fredericksburg, VA 22401 540/899-3588 540/899-2496 (fax)
National Association of Managed Care Physicians	This association is interested in helping physicians cope with the changes wrought by managed care on the independent practitioner. Its meetings usually have a physician focus, but administrators are welcome.	4435 Waterfront Drive, Suite 101 Glen Allen, VA 23060 804/527-1905 804/747-5316 (fax)
National Committee on Quality Assurance	This association provides accreditation services to HMOs and employers. NCQA provides training on a wide variety of quality assurance and plan performance measurement topics throughout the year in locations throughout the U.S.	2000 L Street N.W., Suite 500 Washington, DC 20036 202/955-3500 202/955-3599 (fax)
National IPA Coalition	This trade association provides valuable resources to physician and executive leaders. It is dedicated to enhancing and strengthening physician organizations throughout the country. NIPAC holds two conferences a year on the cutting edge trends and issues on managed care.	1999 Harrison Street, Suite 2750 Oakland, CA 94612 510/267-1999 510/267-8989 (fax) E-mail: info@nipac.org Website: www.nipac.org
The National Managed Health Care Congress	This organization sponsors an annual conference in April, plus regional conferences at other times that are well attended by both vendors and managed care industry professionals. The conference has grown over the last several years to be one of the largest managed care events each year.	71 2nd Avenue, Third Floor Waltham, MA 02143 888/446-6422 617/663-6412 (fax)

Exhibit II–7 Books

Name of Publication	Description	Contact Information
The Capitation Sourcebook	This book provides a comprehensive review of capitation issues and work-arounds to capitation stumbling blocks. It provides the reader with an excellent grounding in at-risk arrangements. Written by Peter Boland, Ph.D.	Jossey-Bass, Publishers 350 Sansome Street San Francisco, CA 94104 415/433-1740 415/433-0499 (fax) E-mail: webperson@ibp.com Website: www.josseybass.com
Making Managed Healthcare Work	This book provides a comprehensive review of managed care successes and their essential elements. It provides an excellent orientation to the best managed care has to offer. Written by Peter Boland, Ph.D.	Aspen Publishers, Inc. 200 Orchard Ridge Drive, Suite 200 Gaithersburg, MD 20878 800/638-8437 301/417-7650 (fax)

INDEX

www.ingramcontent.com/pod-product-compliance
Lightning Source LLC
Chambersburg PA
CBHW060349220326
41598CB00023B/2857